# WOMEN'S MUSCLE & STRENGTH

## Get Lean, Strong, and Confident

Betina Gozo Shimonek

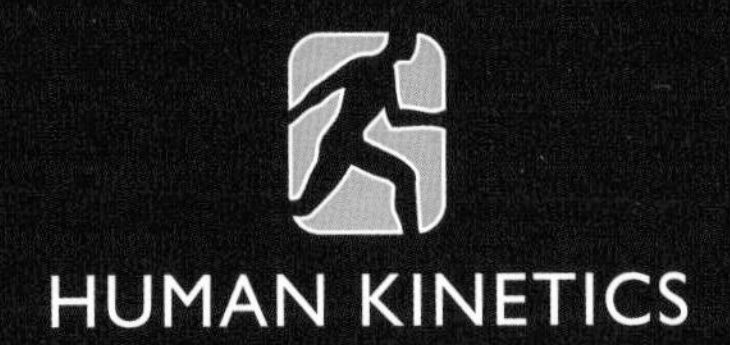

HUMAN KINETICS

**Library of Congress Cataloging-in-Publication Data**

Names: Gozo Shimonek, Betina, 1986- author.
Title: Women's muscle & strength : get lean, strong, and confident / Betina
Gozo Shimonek.
Other titles: Women's muscle and strength
Description: Champaign, IL : Human Kinetics, [2025]
Identifiers: LCCN 2023036556 (print) | LCCN 2023036557 (ebook) | ISBN
9781718217683 (paperback) | ISBN 9781718217690 (epub) | ISBN
9781718217706 (pdf)
Subjects: LCSH: Weight training for women. | Muscle strength. | BISAC:
SPORTS & RECREATION / Bodybuilding & Weightlifting | SPORTS & RECREATION
/ Training
Classification: LCC GV546.6.W64 G69 2025 (print) | LCC GV546.6.W64
(ebook) | DDC 613.7/13082--dc23/eng/20230925
LC record available at https://lccn.loc.gov/2023036556
LC ebook record available at https://lccn.loc.gov/2023036557

ISBN: 978-1-7182-1768-3 (print)



**Senior Acquisitions Editor:** Michelle Earle; **Developmental Editor:** Amy Stahl; **Managing Editor:** Shawn Donnelly; **Copyeditor:** Laura B. Magzis; **Permissions Manager:** Laurel Mitchell; **Senior Graphic Designer:** Joe Buck; **Cover Designer:** Keri Evans; **Cover Design Specialist:** Susan Rothermel Allen; **Photograph (cover):** © Quran Gooch; **Photographs (interior):** © Human Kinetics, unless otherwise noted; **Photo Asset Manager:** Laura Fitch; **Photo Production Specialist:** Amy M. Rose; **Photo Production Manager:** Jason Allen; **Senior Art Manager:** Kelly Hendren; **Illustration:** © Human Kinetics; **Printer:** Versa Press

We thank Crunch Fitness in Champaign, Illinois, for assistance in providing a location for the photo shoot for this book.

Human Kinetics books are available at special discounts for bulk purchase. Special editions or book excerpts can also be created to specification. For details, contact the Special Sales Manager at Human Kinetics.

Printed in the United States of America

10 9 8 7 6 5 4 3 2 1

The paper in this book is certified under a sustainable forestry program.

**Human Kinetics**
1607 N. Market Street
Champaign, IL 61820
USA

*United States and International*
Website: **US.HumanKinetics.com**
Email: info@hkusa.com
Phone: 1-800-747-4457

*Canada*
Website: **Canada.HumanKinetics.com**
Email: info@hkcanada.com

E8921

# WOMEN'S MUSCLE & STRENGTH

# CONTENTS

## PART III Programming for Success

# EXERCISE FINDER

# FOREWORD

I first met Betina in 2015 at a Nike shoot and have had the pleasure of working with her closely ever since. She is a dear friend and mentor and has positively made my life better in so many ways. To say her impact on the wellness industry, specifically with women's strength training, has been hugely positive is an understatement. Betina's passion, enthusiasm, and expertise in training, recovery, and overall wellness—paired with her approachable, supportive, and encouraging nature—are unmatched.

Anyone who has had the privilege of being in the room with Betina knows that her energy and vibrancy fill the entire room. That same enthusiasm and passion meet everything she touches; this is why she is one of my favorite people—I walk away from every interaction feeling inspired.

Strength training for women is so important, and Betina has been a vocal advocate of that for over a decade. She has trained millions of people worldwide, including me, through Nike, Apple Fitness+, LiNE UP With Us, and more—and she's not slowing down. Her mission to make women feel strong, supported, and confident through every age and stage of their lives is beautiful. As a coach and mentor she will challenge you, she'll encourage you, and she'll see you through every step of the path to your goals with a smile on her face.

It's been incredible to watch Betina's journey as a mother and how she has expanded her career into pre- and postpartum training and support for women around the world. In a saturated market of wellness, Betina shines through, offering training and resources that are dynamic and deliver results, backed by years of experience and anchored in education. Most importantly, she focuses on making sure you feel good—not just look good—because confidence is so much more than a reflection in the mirror.

Training with Betina is much more than just exercise. In *Women's Muscle & Strength,* Betina will give you tips, coaching, and motivation to make you feel better in every area of your life. I couldn't be more excited for women around the world to experience her methods and motivation in this book.

—**Kirsty Godso,** Nike Global Trainer

# ACKNOWLEDGMENTS

For my forever supportive husband and biggest cheerleader, Nic: Thank you for always challenging me to be a better coach.

For my firstborn daughter, Aluna, who is a firecracker and future icon for women in sport: You are one of the biggest motivations for me daily.

For my first son, Osa, who was the kicker in my belly while I wrote this book and is forever my Nanay's boy: Thank you for bringing us joy and laughter every day.

*Mahal kita* / I love you!

For anyone who has ever worked out with me: You have touched my life in a special way and always inspire me.

For the whole Human Kinetics team who helped bring this book to life: Thank you for helping me create something to help women everywhere.

*Salamat* / Thank you!

# INTRODUCTION

The gym is intimidating. *What should I do? What equipment should I use? Am I doing this safely? Am I lifting enough? Am I lifting too much*? Whether you are a seasoned pro with weightlifting, an ex-athlete, or just starting out with fitness, you've probably asked yourself one or more of these questions when walking into a gym. The information you see from social media influencers about how they "built a bigger butt" or "got flat abs" is often deceiving, and sometimes so intimidating that most people don't dare to set foot in the gym. Unless you work in the fitness industry (and even sometimes then), listening to coaches sharing the latest technical theory or science factoid is usually boring, confusing, or both. There is a lot of noise out there, and it can be very daunting. You probably picked up this book looking for some answers, tips, or just to drown out the noise of all the conflicting information out there. You're in luck, because I wrote *Women's Muscle & Strength: Get Lean, Strong, and Confident* to do just that. The most important thing to remember is that no matter where you are in your fitness journey, it's exactly that: a journey. No two journeys are the same, but hopefully, with some new, easy-to-implement tools, that journey will be a little less intimidating and a little more fun.

Just like everybody else, I started my journey somewhere too! In 2012, I was playing bass full time in a Top 40 cover band, rocking out for up to three hours, singing and dancing, and swinging my bass guitar around. My bass weighed nearly 12 pounds, and I dropped down into some deep squats with that thing, jumping around on stage with my band. Of course, I was already in pretty good shape. Or so I thought. I remember walking into a gym in Chicago with my roommate, Corey, and heading straight to the stair stepper while she headed to her weekly bootcamp class. Occasionally, I walked over to the "core section" and did a few side bends with some five-pound plates and called it a day. One day, I plucked up the courage to go with Corey to the class. I barely remember what happened in that 45 minutes, other than feeling completely defeated after struggling through the whole class with five-pound dumbbells. I'd be lying if I said I wasn't a little jealous when Corey got through the class with 10-pound dumbbells. I said to myself, *"I can dance around with my bass for three hours! Why can't I survive these 45 minutes and she can!?"*

That's the moment where I could have just given up—turned around and gone right back to my safe space on the stair stepper. Instead of letting that feeling of confusion and jealousy completely take over, I told myself I would keep going back. I was scared at times, especially if Corey couldn't go to class with me and I had to walk in alone. I'd stay in the back and hope the trainer didn't say anything to me. I persevered, and I slowly saw my strength increase. I wasn't ready to pass out after 45 minutes using five-pound weights anymore! Next thing I knew, I confidently used 15 pounds for the entire session.

By this time, not only was I getting stronger, but I started to see my attitude and body change, and not just in the gym. I was making healthier decisions; when my band made our routine gas station stop after a show, I didn't stock up on apple gummy rings and Snickers bars. When we were rocking out at a pub, I chose to not drink as much, if at all. The "wow moment" that showed me how contagious working out is was when my band members started to do squats, push-ups, and planks with me before we went on stage. They would even go with me when we were on the road and had a chance to stop in at a gym. It was making a big impact on my life, not just on me but on the people surrounding me!

While making money playing bass guitar multiple days a week sounds like a dream for any aspiring rock star, I dreamed of getting out. Year after year, we played so many late nights, driving all around the Midwest, taking home nearly nothing for the number of hours we put in. I started to dread some of the shows, playing the same songs over and over. I couldn't quit, though. Not only was this how I made my living, it was how I defined myself! I had played music since I was nine years old, and I was known as the "cool female bass player." Yet, I didn't have enough confidence in myself to know what else I was. As I pushed through show after show, working out was the one thing I always looked forward to. I knew it would make me feel better and stronger, especially after a long weekend of late nights. It started to give me more confidence but also gave me the opportunity to pursue my personal training certification as I started to see a new future for myself.

After months of waking up at 4:30 a.m. to train clients at a gym and riding my bike all across Chicago teaching at multiple studios, I finally felt confident enough to quit. I didn't need the band to define who I was. I loved playing music, but I loved being able to empower other people even more. Because I didn't have much of a sports background or go to college for exercise science, I definitely had a few episodes of imposter syndrome, wondering what gave me the right to tell people how to work out. Thankfully, I had some great mentors, and I used all the extra money I made to take continuing education courses and buy countless strength and exercise science books. I immersed myself in this new world that had once seemed so intimidating to me.

In truth, I wrote this book because I wish someone had given me something like it when I started working out and training clients. I had so many questions. *How do I get the most out of my workouts? Do I have the right form? What the heck is progressive overload or a superset? When should I rest?* As a new trainer, I wanted to know how I should program for my female clients and why I had them doing specific exercises. I wanted to make sure I knew what muscles were being worked and how to help them navigate their bodies and incorporate fitness and exercise into their lives. Through my years of experience, learning from myself as well as my clients, I know that the hardest part is not lifting the weight or correcting form but sticking to a program. My approach is simple and digestible and is meant to be an easy addition to your life, not to take it over. It's designed to help you feel confident with whatever you have in front of you, be it dumbbells or a barbell, or whatever you have in your house. My ultimate goal is to provide the tools for you to be ready and able to adapt to any curveballs life throws your way. I want you to know that it's OK to take a day off if you've had a crazy week or simply want to go with your best friend to that spin class instead of doing your usual routine. I hope this book will be useful to you and maybe even give you that extra push off the stair stepper and into the next phase of your path to fitness.

*Women's Muscle & Strength* is split into three parts. Part I briefly explains some of the basics of how and why a new perspective to strength training is needed. I talk about the benefits you can achieve through consistent strength training along with safety considerations and issues specific to training the female body. I go over some of the phrases you may hear from a trainer or your gym rat friend, like *progressive overload, eccentric,* and more. I've even included a self-assessment to identify your starting point, because watching your progress is one of the best parts!

Part II describes effective exercises organized by movement categories:

- Carry, grip, and antimovement
- Knee dominant and hip dominant
- Horizontal and vertical push
- Horizontal and vertical pull
- Total body and rotational

Don't worry—the terms you may not be familiar with are actually motions you already do every day, in and out of the gym! Plus, you'll see a lot of basic movements like squats, lunges, shoulder presses, rows, and more. I divide the exercises into these movement categories so you can learn how and why to put them together, but you'll also learn what movements are associated with what major muscles, because (let's be real!) I've heard "How do I get a better butt?" countless times in my career. Each movement is illustrated by photos showing correct form, accompanied by detailed instructions. The exercise descriptions include modifications, progressions, variations, safety reminders, and tips because every body is different.

Part III offers four 12-week sample programs based on your goals, the type of equipment you have, and scheduling. The sample programs take real life into account. It isn't always realistic to think everyone should be able to get to the gym every single day. Between jobs, kids, and life in general, you need to choose the routine that will work best for you. Maybe you don't want to give up your weekly cycling or hot yoga class. Or maybe you're like me: a new mom consistently getting short bouts of sleep and having early mornings with a baby! Maybe you only have dumbbells at your house and can't get to the gym at all. Or maybe you're just ready to get after it and are committed to five days a week at to the gym. Regardless, I've got your back. These programs help you figure out what works for you, because fitness shouldn't be "one size fits all."

You've heard some of my story. It's still evolving. No matter where you are on your strength journey, I wrote *Women's Muscle & Strength* to be your workout companion and to help you be and feel successful! I encourage you to keep it handy to refresh your memory or to redirect your routine when life throws something at you.

The gym may be intimidating now, but it doesn't have to be, so let's get stronger!

# PART I

# BECOMING STRONG AND CONFIDENT

# 1

# BENEFITS OF STRENGTH TRAINING FOR WOMEN

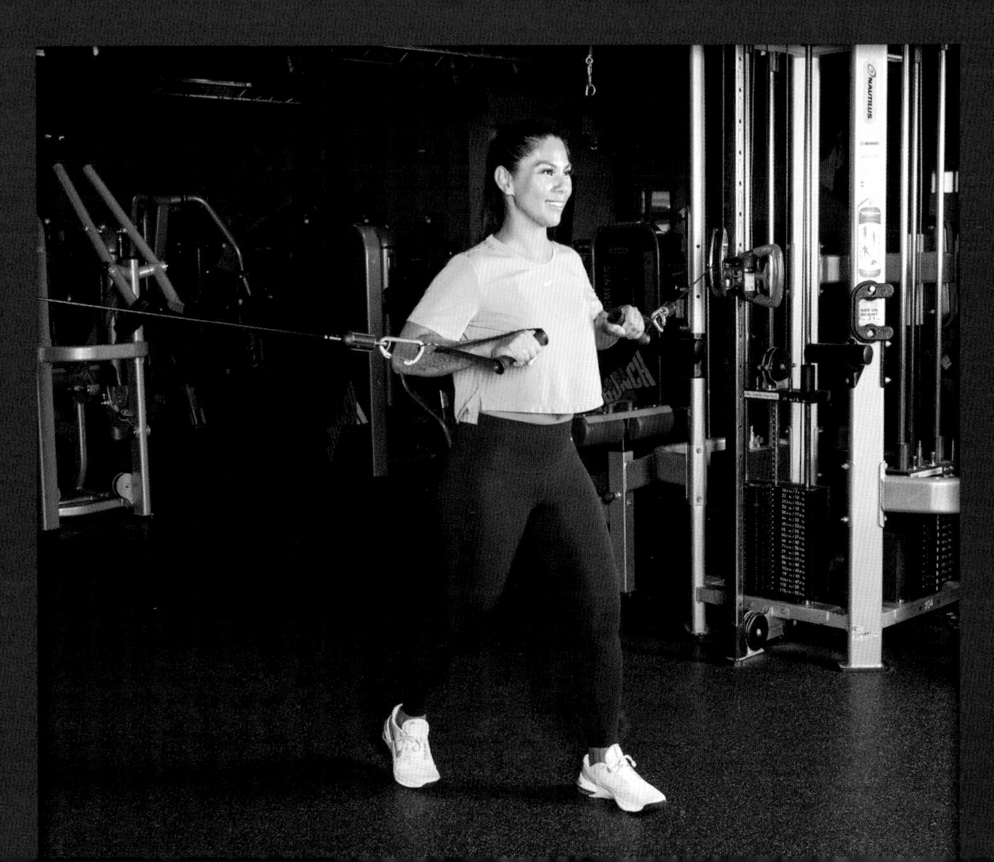

If you've picked up this book, I assume you have an interest in strength training for women and know there are benefits to it. Whether you want to start training because you want to look good or feel better, lifting weights regularly will do both of those things—and so much more! Before I dive into some of the benefits, let's chat about some of the barriers that keep women from strength training.

One of the biggest myths about strength training I still hear after so many years is that lifting weights will make a woman look bulky. How I wish I could scream from every rooftop in the world how untrue this statement can be! Note that I used the word "can." Yes, women who lift weights can become bulky, but it is very difficult and many things come into play. Genetics can have a role, but how you eat and train plays a bigger part in whether you will grow visibly very muscular and bulky. You would have to eat a massive number of calories while following a training program that is meant to bulk you up. None of the programs in this book are intended to do that. Instead, the strength training programs in this book give you the benefits of gaining strength, building muscle, and overall feeling good. We will go over specifics in chapter 4: Getting Started.

Another barrier that keeps women from working out is the gym itself. Some women find gyms intimidating. If you can't relate to this feeling, imagine being a woman who's never worked out before, walking into a space surrounded by lots of unfamiliar equipment, bright lights, and mirrors everywhere, with tons of people moving about from machines to dumbbells. I'm describing a typical "big-box gym" because that is usually the first place that someone who wants to start working out would go. It is likely the lowest cost compared to classes at a fancy boutique studio or a high-end private gym. This brings me to another barrier: cost. It's expensive to equip a home gym, and you must also have enough space for one. This is where the big-box gyms come in. They sell tons of low-cost memberships and often have a sales pitch along these lines: "For less than the monthly cost of a video streaming service, you'll have access to everything a gym has to offer!" But that price might not include a personal trainer or even a simple guide to what you should be doing at the gym. For some gyms, the base fee won't even include classes! Alternatively, if you go to a pricey boutique studio that takes perhaps 20 people per class, you get someone telling you exactly what to do and watching your form, you might get darker, more forgiving lighting, and you probably leave sweating, with tons of endorphins! It's a great investment, but my goal with this book is to help guide you with tools so that you won't need to incur that expense. This way, you can use the inexpensive big-box gym yet still enjoy the benefits of expert training.

Once you leave the intimidation behind, you can reap the benefits of having everything you need at your fingertips! One way to do this is to go to the gym with a friend or family member whom you feel comfortable with. You don't have to work out together, but it's always nice having someone there with you to check in, or even help spot you, when you need it. A lot of gyms offer free classes, and you could attend those and meet people that way, so then you have some familiar faces who can help you feel comfortable getting into a routine. Habits build on each other, so the more often you walk in that door, even if it's only for 20 to 30 minutes, the easier it will get. Overcoming intimidation at the gym is just like strength training itself: The more repetitions you do, the better you become at handling the discomfort and the stronger you'll be. It bears repeating: the more often you walk into that gym and conquer your fear, the more comfortable your body and mind will feel, and the more confident you will feel!

I'll share more details on feeling confident and prepared for the gym in chapter 4, Getting Started. In the remainder of this chapter, I discuss the various benefits of strength training.

# SOME STRENGTH TRAINING BENEFITS

From feeling physically stronger to managing mental health better, the benefits to strength training are virtually endless. For women specifically, strength training can also increase the ability to cope with the different stages of life, like pregnancy and menopause. In addition, strength training can result in better sleep and help regulate the effects of various hormones. Whether you want to find out why it's best for you or you want to explain the benefits to someone else, let's dig in.

## Physical Health

The physical benefits are probably the most popular and widely known benefit of strength training. Strength training not only helps build muscle to help you appear leaner and more toned, but building muscle increases your metabolic rate throughout the day, sometimes up to 72 hours after you're done training. This is significant compared to the number of calories that you burn during cardiovascular exercises. More often than not, when doing cardio, like running or dancing, the number of calories you burn may be a lot more than calories burned during a weight training session, but you burn those active calories only during that time. With strength training, you're likely to continue burning calories after your workout, especially if it was a particularly intense one. So yes, you will burn calories even while you're sitting on the couch!

Besides the calorie burn during and after strength training, you're also building a stronger body to help overall functionality and activities of daily life. You'll be able to move better and more comfortably throughout the day. From the simplest tasks, like carrying groceries or moving furniture around the house, to the extreme of helping move your car if it breaks down, you'll be thankful for your strength training. The act of weight training can also help with something called *proprioception*, which is your awareness of your body in space. The more purposeful you are with moving and strengthening your muscles, the better you are able to move throughout your world!

For someone who plays sports, whether professionally or recreationally, strength training can increase power, speed, endurance, and stamina, as well as help reduce the risk of injury and prevent muscle strain. There aren't many professional athletes with long, successful careers who don't make weight training a big part of what they do. If playing tennis or pickleball is something you like to do for fun every weekend, then adding a strength routine is optimal for longevity. A regular strength routine has also been shown to help manage symptoms and decrease the risk of some diseases and conditions, such as osteoporosis, osteoarthritis, obesity, diabetes, and more.

## Mental Health

Mental health is now more commonly talked about than in years past. There is a good correlation between a healthy relationship with exercise and a strong sense of mental health. There are many studies that have shown that physical activity can improve mental health, anxiety, and depression symptoms. There's a popular movie in which the law student character points out, "Exercise gives you endorphins. Endorphins make you happy. Happy people just don't shoot their husbands; they just don't!" (She was speaking of a popular fitness instructor accused of murdering her husband, but—spoiler alert!—didn't.) In my many years in the fitness industry, I'd agree that most of the instructors and trainers I know don't carry a lot of negative energy. Because working out releases endorphins and dopamine, or as some call it, "the happy hormone," it can help you manage daily. There are also some other positive effects of strength training for your brain, like increasing neuroplasticity and preventing neurodegeneration. What?! Yes, studies have suggested that a regular strength training routine in combination with good sleep and nutrition can improve memory, focus, and other cognitive skills.

As I mentioned, making a habit out of going to the gym can increase your confidence. Building that confidence may help with mental health related to insecurities too. I've always believed that the good vibes you get when you feel yourself getting stronger and see your physical progress seep into other aspects of life. I've had clients who, after increasing their exercise, feel more confident giving a presentation at work or talking with new people. Exercise can help you manage so many different life stressors. However, it is important to note that if you are suffering from depression or other mental health issues and are not seeing any improvement through exercise, it is highly recommended to see a therapist or doctor of psychiatry.

## Aging

I've worked with a number of older clients who say exercising makes them generally feel better, even if they're not slinging around barbells and kettlebells. Strength training can be defined as any form of resistance, including body weight! When you challenge your bones with any kind of weight-bearing exercise, you are putting temporary stress on them, which helps those bones become stronger over time. As we age, we lose bone density and muscle mass, but weight-bearing exercise can help combat various issues, such as developing osteoporosis, loss of balance or coordination, or the simple risk of being unable to perform everyday activities—even small amounts of strength training can be highly beneficial over many years. No matter what age you are, it's never too late to make strength training a habit.

## Menstrual, Premenopausal, and Hormonal Health

Women have a menstrual cycle and most have the ability to grow and carry a human or two (or more!). Women also have a wide range of hormones.

As previously mentioned, exercise can help increase dopamine, "the happy hormone," which in turn decreases stress. During a woman's menstrual cycle, that dopamine can help regulate some emotions that come with other hormones. In my years of training women, many of them have reported feeling fewer aches and pains from cramps thanks to a regular strength training routine. If you are not feeling up for an intense workout, you can adapt your programming (or the weight that you are using). If you do not have any debilitating injuries or soreness, it can be beneficial to get a session in, even if you have to modify the exercises. Lots of women ask when the best time to exercise is during the menstrual cycle. During your period, there is an increase of inflammation in your body, which is why a lot of women don't feel good during this time. The same goes for the premenstrual phase, the time right before your period, when all the cravings come in and your body is preparing for the imminent inflammation. Directly before your premenstrual time is the start of your luteal phase, when your progestogen hormone is released. Progestogen is a catabolic hormone that drives the breakdown of tissue, so you may notice more soreness or your workouts may feel more intense than usual at this time. Put another way, that breakdown of muscle is more likely during this phase because of the progesterone release. As far as feeling good and managing the inflammation and breakdown of muscle, this is where nutrition and managing your sleep comes in. So when is the best time to exercise during your menstrual cycle? The general answer is, any time during the cycle is a good time to exercise. You'll always reap the benefits of exercise, as long as you're feeling up for it! You may even find that you have more energy after you're done. I've always been a big advocate of tracking your periods and how you're feeling. This will boost your awareness of your cycle and help you learn how to manage it with your nutrition and workouts.

For women nearing menopause, getting your heart rate up for at least half an hour every day can help boost estrogen levels. This can help manage the symptoms of menopause since they are in part driven by the imbalance and decline of estrogen.

## Sleep Health

Lastly, lifting heavy weights can increase the growth hormone and serotonin, which both help with sleep. Sleep and the growth hormone go hand in hand. The more you sleep, the better your growth hormone regulates so that your body can recover and restore itself. Serotonin has been shown to help with regulating your circadian rhythms, getting to sleep, and waking up at a regular time. In order to get your sleep in check, it's important to go to sleep around the same time each evening to avoid being overtired. Babies are such a good example of the purest form of a regulated circadian rhythm. Our daughter sleeps best if we put her to bed around 7:30 p.m. She will sleep a full 12 hours and wake up around 7:30 a.m. the next day. If we put her to bed any later than 7:30, she usually wakes up earlier, sometimes as early as 6 a.m.! Getting on that regular schedule is important, and your weight training routine will help. Plus, lifting weights will make you just the right amount of tired, just like it gives you the right amount of energy. Similar to tracking your periods, tracking your workouts in correlation with your sleep can be helpful to see what works for you.

## Pregnancy

You may have heard something like "You can do what you always were doing when it comes to exercise, but you shouldn't try anything new" once you become pregnant. While this is somewhat true, it's also not quite accurate. If you haven't been exercising prior to pregnancy, it doesn't mean you should not exercise at all once you become pregnant. There are some restrictions, and we'll go through those in the next chapter. But actually pregnancy is a good time to begin strength training under the supervision of a prenatal specialist. There are a ton of benefits to working out during pregnancy, as long as you have a healthy pregnancy and you've been cleared by your doctor or midwife.

In summary, incorporating strength training into your life has myriad benefits, among them improving activities of daily life, getting better sleep, and boosting energy throughout the day. Women who exercise during pregnancy have also reported fewer aches and pains from the changes in their bodies, especially the changes in center of gravity. While there are many benefits to the woman, there are also some benefits to the baby. Some studies suggest that exercising while pregnant can improve the baby's ability to manage the stress of labor, and it can also benefit the baby after the birth by reducing the chance of diabetes or other metabolic diseases. Pregnancy is a pivotal time in a woman's life, when so many changes are happening in their bodies. Doing what you can to keep your body strong and able to cope with the changes and stresses is important.

This chapter was meant to reiterate the beauty that strength training has for anyone, especially women. I know that training can help a woman tremendously in so many aspects of her life, and I hope that after learning all the benefits you can see how everything ties together. Better nutrition, regulating sleep, managing stress, and incorporating mindfulness—exercise can help strengthen all those things and make living a lot easier and more joyful!

# 2

# SAFETY DURING STRENGTH TRAINING

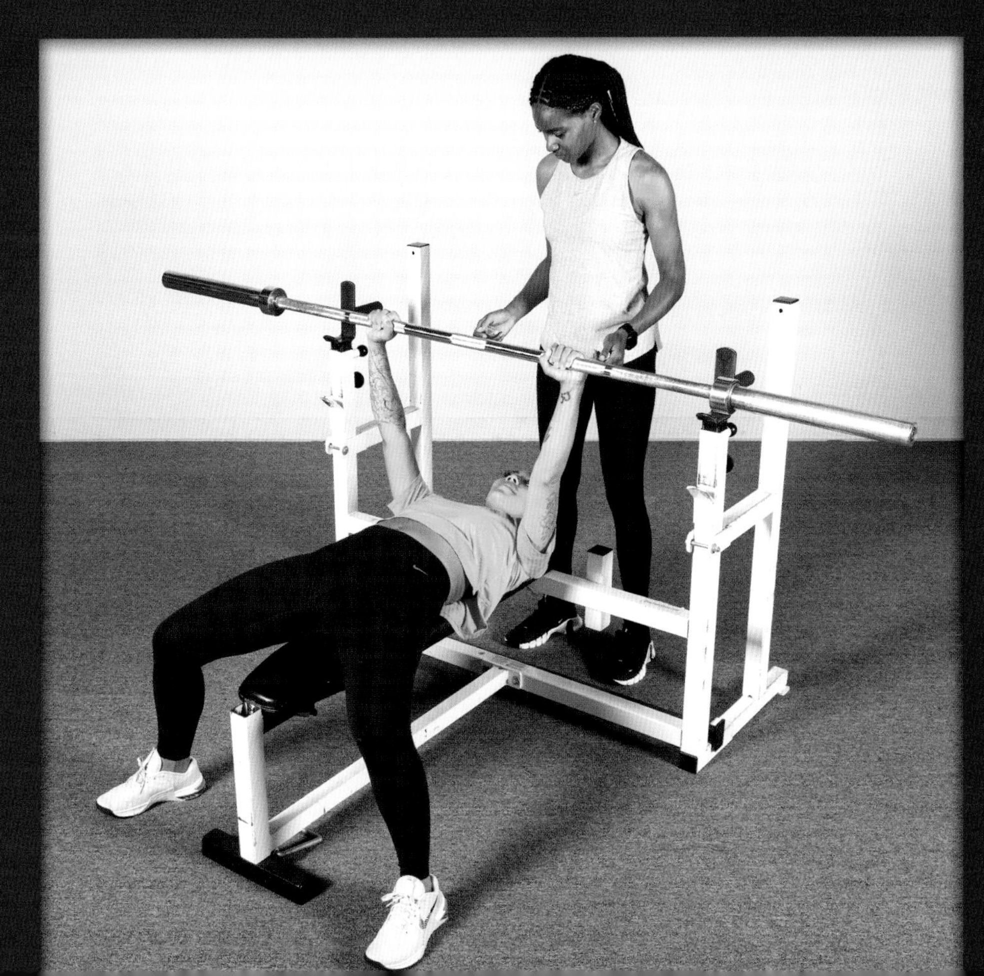

Something I hear a lot as a coach is the question of how safe strength training is. Repeatedly picking up a heavy weight and putting it back down may seem risky, but if you use proper form, it can minimize the risk of injury for a lot of everyday activities, such as picking up a bag of groceries. This chapter discusses ways to exercise more safely.

## KEEPING YOUR WORKOUTS SAFER

When I first began working out, I always found it helpful and encouraging to work out with someone else for motivation and safety. Generally, it's a good idea to lift weight when there is someone else in the room, in case of any accidents. This can mean a public place like a gym or a private space when another person is there. (If you are new to working out, this may be intimidating, but chapter 4 goes over some tips to help you feel more confident and comfortable.)

In addition to the need to have someone present when you lift weight in case of an emergency, there are some exercises for which you'll occasionally need someone to "spot" you, particularly when you are challenging yourself with a lot of weight. What does having someone spot you actually entail? Depending on the exercise—usually a squat or chest press—the person stands behind you, ready to assist, in case you are not able to move the weight for your last rep. Your spotter is there for support and motivation and may just help guide you as you rerack the weight or put it down. You want someone who can hold the weight they are spotting for you; otherwise, you may be in a dangerous situation if you actually need them. It's not uncommon to ask someone you do not know at the gym to give you a quick spot. Keep in mind that this person does not need to touch you and may not need to touch the weight. I will mention in the exercise descriptions when it is recommended to have a spotter, but it's generally OK to ask for help or a spotter any time you feel you need one.

## PROPER REST AND RECOVERY

Once you get used to strength training and you're seeing yourself get stronger, it's very easy to get excited about how strong you're getting. This goes for any exercise. The endorphins are real! You are in a good mood, you are feeling super motivated, and you're wondering, Who is this person who's *excited* about working out? This is a great feeling, of course, but don't get carried away just yet. You must be mindful of trying to progress too quickly, such as by increasing the weight too quickly or doing too many workouts back to back, without proper rest and recovery. In strength training, it is important to allow adequate rest periods between each workout set. Typically, 30 seconds to 2 minutes is necessary so that your muscles can reset, recover, and be ready for the next set.

You can avoid progressing too fast by following a program and tracking the weight that you are using for each exercise. Following this practice can help you "progressively overload" (read more about this in chapter 3). While it is very exciting to see yourself lifting heavy weight, know that when you lift, you are actually creating little tears in your muscles that then repair themselves to get stronger. That is why rest and sleep are needed. You cannot trick your body out of poor sleep. Getting enough sleep is one of the most important things you can do for yourself. If you had a challenging workout followed by a few consecutive nights of poor sleep, it may be a good idea to back off from a workout and skip it that day to allow your body more time to recover. When you do not allow your body to recover and your muscles to repair, you can also experience symptoms of overtraining. Overtraining is simply what happens when your body cannot recover from what you are asking it to do . The symptoms of overtraining can be prolonged general fatigue, a plateau or decrease in your progress, an inability to relax, increased melancholy or anger, or a combination of these indicators.

## INJURY AND EXERCISE

An injury can be a good *reason* not to exercise, but it's not necessarily a good *excuse*. If you have an upper-body injury and it's possible to safely work your lower body, then do it—and vice versa. But be sure to get clearance from a medical professional before working out if you are seriously injured, are recovering from an injury, or have had any recent major surgeries. When your doctor has cleared you to exercise, I highly recommend physical or occupational therapy to ensure you are moving well and have no overcompensations due to your injury or surgery that can be exacerbated by exercise. I'm talking here about physical therapy after an injury, yet a lot of the work physical therapists do with their patients is more mental than physically strenuous. If you have a nagging knee or shoulder issue, you may find some benefit in a few physical therapy sessions. I've always been fond of physical therapists who understand strength training. This knowledge helps tremendously when you're transitioning back into strength training after an injury because the physical therapist may give you movements that can help you with the specific training you want to do after your rehab. As with strength exercises, the repetitions of rehab exercises you learn in physical or occupational therapy can help your body move better and improve its strength.

## PREGNANCY AND POSTPARTUM

As a prenatal- and postpartum-certified trainer who's had two pregnancies, I always advocate for safely exercising during these special times. As a reminder, it's always important to check with your doctor or midwife to make sure that exercise is right for you during this time. Your doctor or midwife is an advocate for the health of you and your baby, and their job is to guide your general health and wellness throughout the journey. They are not trained in what specific strength training or pelvic floor exercises you should be doing. When it comes to specific exercise and movements, guidance from a prenatal or postpartum strength-training specialist is recommended.

During pregnancy and the postpartum stage, you may want to see a pelvic floor physical therapist. It's a common misconception that during pregnancy, you should do a million Kegels (pelvic floor contractions) to "strengthen your pelvic floor." But during birth your pelvic floor must relax to allow your baby through the birth canal. A pelvic floor physical therapist can assess if you need to strengthen your pelvic floor and can help you to coordinate your breath with pelvic floor contractions. They can also help with labor preparation and prepare you for a good postpartum recovery. When it comes to the postpartum experience, you may hear women joke about peeing their pants when they run or jump. While this is very common, it is a sign of dysfunction in your pelvic floor. The pelvic floor physical therapist can help with any prolapse issues and ensure that you are engaging your pelvic floor properly. Pelvic floor physical therapy isn't just for prenatal and postpartum training, though. Some people have incontinence issues or have trouble engaging their transverse abdominals. Understandably, this can be frustrating and can even keep someone from working out! Know that even though it is a sign of dysfunction, after just a few sessions with a pelvic floor specialist, you may be on your way to more comfortable workouts!

As mentioned in the first chapter, it is OK to start exercising while pregnant. Each pregnant athlete is unique, and so I recommend finding a local trainer who is a prenatal specialist to help guide you. Here are some general guidelines that may help you along the way. During the first trimester, your body changes a lot, especially if it is your first time being pregnant. Most women have some form of nausea, with some worse than others. I think this is a good time to remember that it's OK to take a break from exercising if you need extra sleep in the morning or a lunchtime nap. Having gone through two pregnancies as a fitness professional, I can proudly share I did more napping than working out in my first trimester. Nevertheless, it is advisable to get some movement into your day, even just an easy walk outside.

In general, and always complying with your medical professional's advice, you can proceed with exercise as normal in your first trimester, but you should generally not take up a new sport or a physical activity you've never tried. With your regular exercise routine, some adjustments may be needed. For instance, as your body changes, it may start to get uncomfortable to lie face down, so you may want to modify certain exercises. Additionally, the levels of the hormone relaxin during pregnancy are higher. Because of this, there will be more laxity in your ligaments, especially in your hips and pelvis, so avoid overstretching and be cautious of any single-leg movements or anything that may put you off balance. I encourage a lot of stability exercises throughout pregnancy, especially for your hips, and strength training can help with that. There are little things you can do to keep yourself safer, like avoiding high-impact exercises that have a high risk for injury, and squatting down and then rolling to your side before lying down on the ground. Most core exercises that involve lying on your back—for instance, crunches or anything involving extending or lifting your legs—should not be done until after childbirth and you have been cleared to exercise by your healthcare provider. The focus for core work should be breathing exercises and exercises that keep a neutral spine while adding a little movement. This is to avoid any extra abdominal pressure and thus prevent coning due to diastasis recti, or the splitting of your abdominals. Extreme rotation of your shoulders and hips should also be avoided, but some basic upper-back and total body rotational movements are welcome, as long as your hips and shoulders stay in line—you don't want to "wring out" your belly!

During your second trimester, you regain some energy and feel ready to conquer workouts again. Take this time to ease back into workouts, especially if you weren't able to exercise much during your first trimester. Continuing with strength training is a good way to feel strong during this time, allowing for adjustments for your growing body whenever needed. It is not a time to lift the heaviest weight you have but instead to focus on feeling good and maintaining strength as your body changes. In your third trimester you may notice you'll have to make the most adjustments, such as not lying on your back for an extended period of time. If needed, you can always prop yourself up with a pillow for an adjustment to an exercise.

To be clear, I don't want you to feel like pregnancy means no intense workouts. I'm a big advocate for women maintaining their strength via high-intensity exercise as long as it feels comfortable. But as with any exercise, it's always worth asking if the risk is higher than the reward. For example, if you love to do Olympic-style lifting, the barbell clean may not be worth doing as your belly grows because the risk of injury outweighs the benefit of the exercise. Some things can wait until you're ready in the postpartum period!

I am more vocal about how much more cautious you should be after childbirth than during the pregnancy. You either gave birth vaginally or had a cesarean. Both are major events that your body needs time to recover from. Some postpartum women are able to take easy walks on the day of birth, while some may have to wait a week or two. The most important thing is that you wait for your doctor or midwife to clear you to exercise, which is typically not until the 6-week postpartum appointment. Before then, you may incorporate easy breathing and pelvic floor contractions (Kegels), and perhaps some gentle stretching. When your health care provider clears you to exercise, it does not mean you jump right into what you were doing before. It's crucial to ease back into everything, especially weight training. After giving birth, you can restart core activation and breath coordination with movement. Lifting too heavy too quickly can lead to pelvic organ prolapse or diastasis recti, so it's important to go slowly as you make your way back into training. If you are still not sure what kind of program or workouts you should be doing, work with a postpartum specialist to design a program specially designed for you during this period.

These safety precautions aren't meant to scare you away from exercising—they're here to empower you and make you feel confident! Proper recovery may help you reach your goals faster, and getting an injury taken care of by the proper health care provider may shorten the time it takes to heal. The next chapter covers one of my favorite things to teach as a coach. We'll go over some basic movement anatomy and look at some of the equipment you see in the gym. Let's get up and go!

# 3

# EQUIPMENT AND MOVEMENT FOUNDATIONS

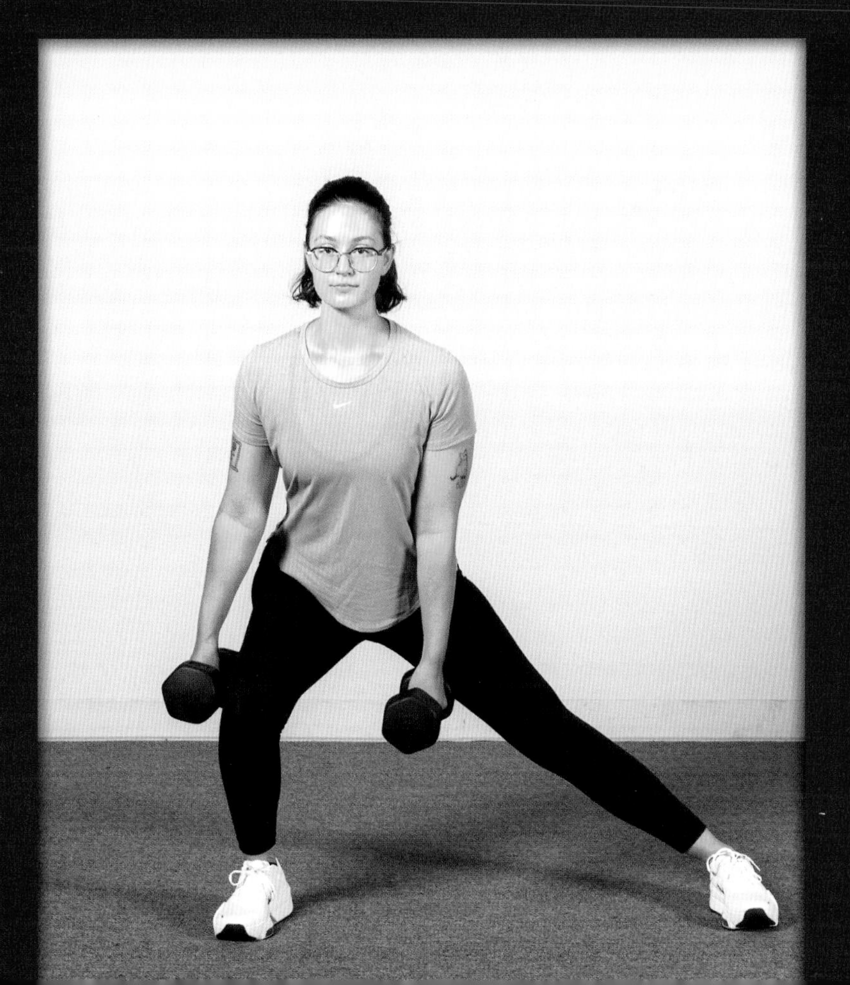

You will find at the gym many pieces of equipment used for strength training, but in this chapter I look closely at the specific equipment you need for the exercises and programs in this book and how you can set yourself up for success at home, if you choose to work out there. It can be overwhelming when you walk into a gym not knowing where to start or what piece of equipment to pick up first. For the exercises in this book, the free-weights section with dumbbells is where you'll spend a lot of your time. When it comes to building your own set at home, you may have limited space, but you also want to get the most out of your workouts. This chapter gives you the knowledge you need to feel more comfortable with the equipment you will use and gives you basic anatomy and fitness-jargon lessons to help you understand strength training and how it pertains to the programs in this book.

# EQUIPMENT

When I think of a typical gym, I imagine rows of treadmills and stair steppers, one or two squat racks, and a big row of dumbbells with a few adjustable benches. Any of the programs in this book can be done in this setting, but two programs can also be done at home. In this book, you will not use any large, fixed-range-of-motion machines, like a leg press, leg extension, or seated chest fly. These machines offer a multitude of benefits, but the focus in these programs is on using free weights like those highlighted in this section. (Chapter 4 details what you need for each program.)

## Barbell

Most gyms have a regular Olympic barbell that is about 45 pounds (20.4 kg). Some gyms may even have a barbell geared toward women that is about 35 pounds (15.9 kg) and a little smaller in circumference, for women's hands, but about the same length as a "standard" barbell. Additionally, you may find a training bar, which is typically shorter and about 15 pounds (6.8 kg). These are typically used to teach the movement pattern of Olympic lifts, like a clean or overhead snatch, but you aren't able to load the bar with a lot of weight. If you are going to purchase a barbell for yourself, the women's barbell would be my recommendation to start. You'll also need two clips and a foam pad that goes around the bar for hip thrusts. You may see the foam pad advertised as a barbell pad for squats, but I don't recommend using them for that. While it may provide relief for your shoulders as the weight is sitting on them, it allows for one more barrier of contact between your shoulders and the barbell. This can possibly cause the bar to be off balance from your shoulders, or even roll back, causing you to drop the bar. (Using a spotter might alleviate this issue.)

At most gyms, you'll find a variety of plates to add to the bar. If you'd like to purchase some for yourself, be aware that the price tag will grow as you get stronger. The heavier the plates are, the pricier they will get! A good place to start with plates is: (2) 2.5 pound (1.13 kg); (2) 5 pound (2.26 kg); (2) 10 pound (4.53 kg); (2) 15 pound (6.80 kg); and (2) 25 pound (11.33 kg). Ideally, you would also have a squat rack, which we'll dive into next.

## Squat Rack

You'll find a squat rack at most gyms. A squat rack comprises two steel stands with pins that allow you to adjust the height where the bar will be racked. You may also find another rack that looks similar called a Smith machine, where the barbell is fixed on the rack. Either option can work, but the free weights on a regular squat rack will allow you to move freely through your own range of motion, recruiting more muscles. A squat rack for a home gym can be pricey and also take up a lot of space, but there are some that are foldable for a smaller footprint.

## Dumbbells

There are many types of dumbbells, and most you find at any gym will work for the programs in this book. You can choose from a few options if you want to purchase dumbbells for home use. I recommend having a set of dumbbells from 5 pounds (2.26 kg) to 30 pounds (13.60 kg) for the at-home programs. If you have the budget, it would be beneficial to have multiple sets of dumbbells that go up in increments of 2.5 pounds (1.13 kg). This is so that you are not significantly increasing weight from one week to the next, but if you have to do that, there is a range of repetition schemes that you can adapt as necessary. There are also adjustable dumbbells you can find that can go from 5 pounds (2.26 kg) all the way up to 100 pounds (45.35 kg)! As with individual dumbbells, the more expandable weights you add onto adjustable ones, the pricier the dumbbells get. Adjustable dumbbells take up less space, but they do have disadvantages: Some may require extra steps to adjust the weight and this can be frustrating if you are doing a superset or circuit that needs different weight for different exercises.

## Kettlebells

In the programs included in this book, kettlebells aren't necessary, but they can be used for some of the exercises in place of the dumbbells. For example, a goblet squat with a dumbbell can be replaced with a kettlebell. They can be very beneficial because of their shape and weight distribution, emulating the load of heavy everyday items such as a bag of groceries. Holding a kettlebell feel different from holding a dumbbell because of their different shapes. If you are doing a dumbbell exercise in the rack position, you will have to use a different grip when using a kettlebell, with the kettlebell's weight resting on your forearms. This can put more pressure on your forearms and make the exercise more challenging. More information on the rack position for kettlebells can be found in the exercise descriptions.

## Bench

You'll need an adjustable bench that lies flat and also adjusts to a seated position, which you will find at most gyms. If you have one that does not adjust to a seated position, you can still make it work; simply sit upright at the end of the bench. However, the seated position on a bench with an adjustable section allows for more back support. Find one that feels comfortable and supportive! You should always make sure the bench is locked in once it's adjusted, so that it does not move while you are training.

## Pull-Up Bar

A pull-up bar can be found in different setups at a gym. It can be part of a squat rack, part of the functional trainer cable machine (see next section), or it can be on its own, hung on a wall or freestanding. Any of these options will work, as long as it is anchored safely and there is a box nearby that you can step on to reach the bar. If you're buying a pull-up bar for your home, look for one that doesn't take up a lot of space and can hook into a doorway or be bolted into the wall.

## Functional Trainer Cable Machine

Unless you have a big space for your home gym, this isn't an ideal piece of equipment to purchase for at-home use because of its large footprint. When this book was written, cable machines with a small footprint were becoming more common, but they are usually more expensive. If you want to buy a cable machine for these programs, look for one that allows you to adjust the angle and height of the anchor. Most have pins that adjust to a desired weight, but there is one that uses air compression. As an alternative, inexpensive superbands can take the place of a few of the cable machine exercises in these programs. See the next section for more on these.

## Superbands

Superbands are rubber latex bands that measure about 40 inches in circumference (about 102.6 cm) but vary in thickness. The thicker the band is, the more resistance there is, and the thinner they are, the less resistance. Superband exercises can be used in place of some of the cable machine exercises in this program, as long as you have a solid anchor where you can attach the band. These bands can also help with assisted pull-ups. I recommend starting with a variety of 4 different band widths, including 3/4 inches (1.9 cm), 1-1/4 inches (3.175 cm), 1-3/4 inches (4.445 cm), and 2.5 inches (6.35 m). If you are using a superband in place of a cable machine with an attachment, you will simply use the band as your handle, finding the grip around the band that feels good for you.

## ATTACHMENTS

You can find a variety of attachments at the gym for a functional trainer cable machine. The ones you use in this program are single handles, double handles, an ankle strap, and a bar for pull-downs with both arms. The attachment you need is specified in the exercise descriptions. You may find other types of attachments, like a rope handle, which may be substituted for single or double handles if you are unable to find them.

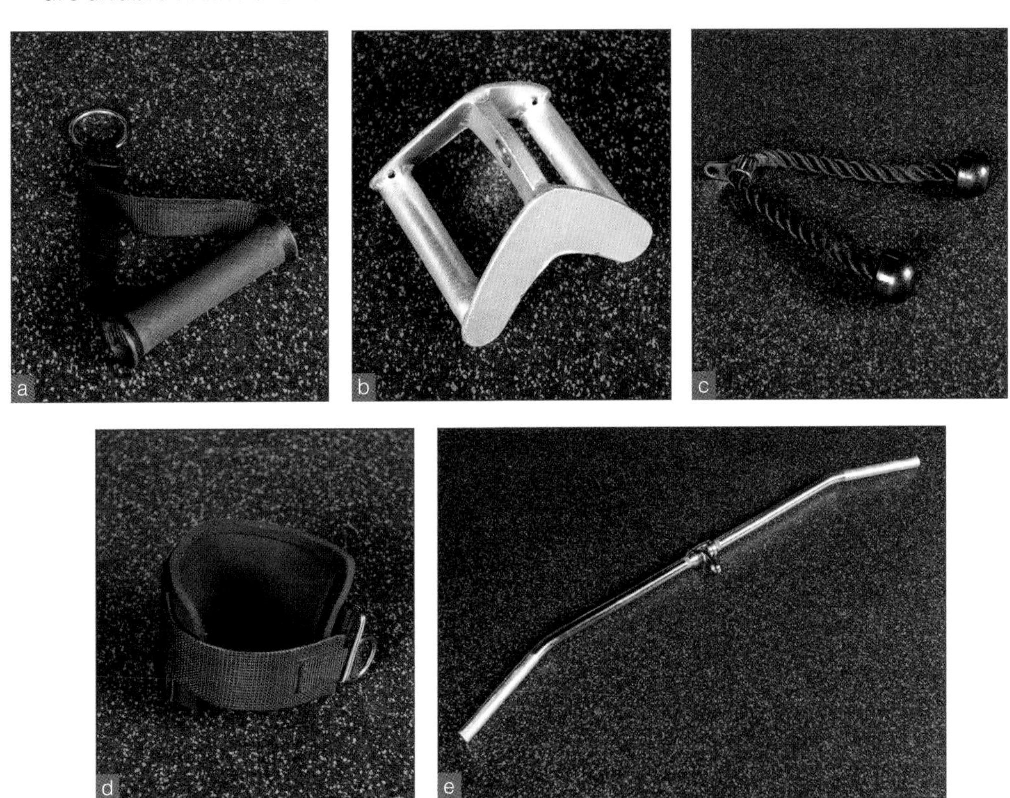


Examples of cable machine attachments: (*a*) single handle, (*b*) double handle, (*c*) double rope handle, (*d*) ankle strap, and (*e*) pull-down bar.

# PLANES OF MOTION AND ANATOMICAL DIRECTIONS

When we move in everyday life, we move in many dimensions, or planes of motion. Planes are described by which direction they pass through, and the plane of motion is the space in which the motion occurs: sagittal, frontal, and transverse (see figure 3.1). When you see an athlete move in multidirectional sports, like soccer or basketball, they are moving in these different planes at any given moment. In strength training, it's very common to see most exercises done in the sagittal plane, where there is a lot of opportunity to move a lot of weight. However, it is important to train in every plane of motion, including multiple planes at once, to help reduce the risk of injury, improve stability and balance, and increase overall performance and functionality. The more you train in varied planes of motion both unilaterally and bilaterally, the better your awareness of your body's motion in space will be.

In this section, I use visuals like walls or a tube. I'd like you to know that these are examples that are meant to generally help you picture the movement done in the specific plane. If you break down every movement of an exercise, there will technically be multiple motions happening in different planes, but most exercises refer to the main movement or prime mover of the exercise. Those are what I reference in the following. Let's dig in deeper to what all of these terms mean.

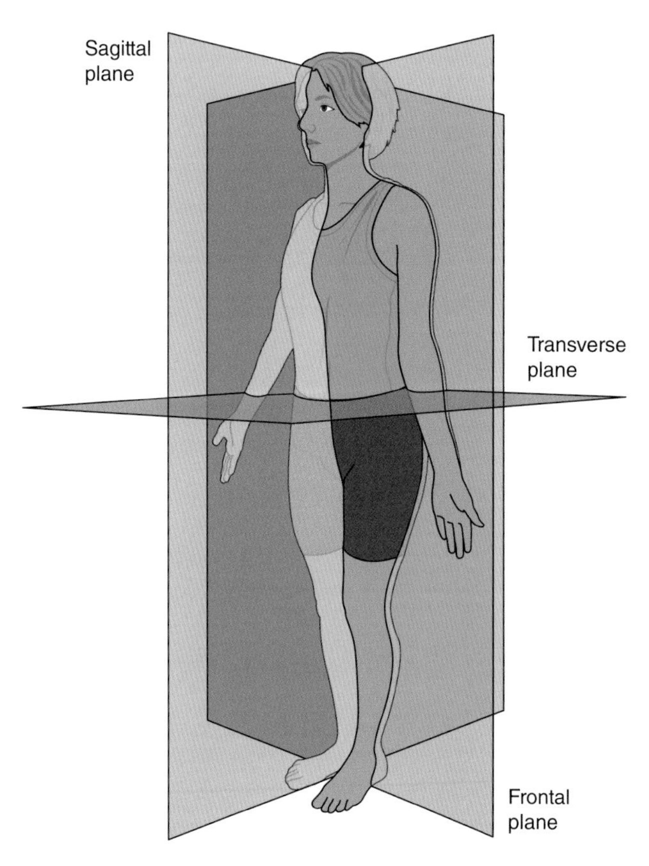


**FIGURE 3.1** Movement planes of the human body: sagittal plane divides the body into left and right; transverse plane separates the head from the feet, and frontal plane splits body from front and back.

## Sagittal Plane

The sagittal plane is a vertical plane that splits the body into left and right sides, and the motion that occurs in this plane is typically forward and back movements, or flexion and extension of the spine, hips, knees, and elbows. Pretend you are stuck in between two walls on the left and right side of your body. Most of the exercises you can do in between these walls are in the sagittal plane, like forward or reverse lunges, biceps curls, front raises, push-ups, and even crunches or back extensions. The bigger and more conventional lifts, like chest press, bent row, front or back squat, and deadlifts are in the sagittal plane. These exercises are all lifts that most people feel the most stable performing, so more opportunities exist in these exercises to add more weight to increase strength.

## Frontal Plane

Now pretend that those same two walls are in front and behind you; the movement you can do in between these walls is likely in the frontal plane. Like the sagittal plane, this is another vertical plane, but it splits the body from front and back, with motion occurring laterally (side to side) or a motion moving toward or away from the midline of the body. Movements like a side bend, lateral lunge, lateral raises, or jumping jacks are all in the frontal plane. If you're in a side plank or side-lying position, a leg lift would also be moving in the frontal plane. These exercises help you work many muscles that support the prime movers of lifts like a squat or chest press, and they help you move more efficiently through everyday movements like walking or running.

## Transverse or Horizontal Plane

The transverse plane is split into top and bottom halves, and typically the motions are rotational or twisting movements. Imagine you are stuck in a tube, and most of the movements that can be done to take space in the tube are in this plane. You can rotate your head side to side, pivot your feet so you rotate your whole body left or right, or twist the upper part of your body to face left or right. This also includes internally or externally rotating your limbs like your arms or legs. The transverse plane is not limited to this small tube, though. If you are doing a type of lunge where you step forward or backward to a diagonal, this would also be movement in the transverse plane.

Some exercises in the transverse plane may feel unconventional or unfamiliar, but rotation is essential for better everyday movement, injury resilience, and increasing your proprioception. Try to think of how many times a day you move in the transverse plane, like when you're putting on your seatbelt or putting away dishes on a corner shelf. You do it often! In these programs, you'll find a combination of core stability movements in conjunction with transverse exercises. This is so you can apply the stability to these complex movements in both your training and your daily life!

### Multiplanar

Multiplanar movements are when you combine two or all three of the planes of motion. This is what you are already doing every day, as when you pick something up off the floor or reach for something in the back seat of your car. Some exercise examples of this combine the sagittal and transverse plane into one move, like a forward lunge with a rotation, and some combine all three planes with a move like a full body woodchop. When it comes to strength training, you typically won't see these movements with really heavy loads, because an added level of stability and coordination is required.

### Bilateral

"Bilateral" in exercise science refers to both sides of your body working simultaneously in the same plane of motion, typically in the sagittal plane. A squat with both feet planted in the sagittal plane or an overhead press with both arms starting and ending in the same position and moving at the same time are examples of this type of exercise. You could also say you are in a "bilateral stance," which means both feet are planted in in the sagittal plane, or a "bilateral overhead press," referring to both arms pressing up at the same time instead of alternately.

### Unilateral

"Unilateral" generally refers to using one side of the body at a time, but it can mean many different things. Standing on one leg, moving one side of your body only, or holding load on one side are all unilateral. A one-arm overhead press can be referred to as a "unilateral overhead press," but it can also be considered unilateral if you are alternating sides. Similarly, "unilateral stance" may refer to a single-leg Romanian deadlift and standing on one leg is a "unilateral squat." A lunge is considered a unilateral exercise because of its single-sided nature of movement, whether you're alternating or staying on one side.

## MUSCLE CONTRACTIONS

Every movement you make in the gym or in daily life has some combination of an eccentric, isometric, or concentric muscle contraction. In the programs in this book, I incorporate a specific tempo or time limit for each contraction, so it's important to understand at what phase that time or tempo exists. While there are benefits to isolating the contractions as their own exercise, it's important to train all three phases of the contractions to move optimally.

## Isometric

An isometric contraction is when the muscle is contracting and actively fighting gravity or weight, but not lengthening or shortening. Sometimes this contraction is simply called a "hold." When you are at the bottom of a squat and holding it there, that is an isometric contraction. There is no change in the muscle length at that point, but there is an active contraction. If you are simply standing at the top of your squat and not holding a weight, there is no tension or force, so it's unlikely that an isometric contraction is happening. If you are about to do a squat, holding some dumbbells in a rack position, there will be an isometric contraction in your arms but not in your legs. If you lower down and hold about halfway into your squat with your dumbbells still in a rack position, there will be another isometric contraction, in your legs, in addition to your arms. (Extra burn!) Another example of an isometric contraction is a plank or push-up position. In the top portion of a push-up an isometric contraction happens because gravity causes your core muscles and shoulder stabilizers to fire up. An isometric hold at the end range of a movement is something I commonly add into the first phase of a strength program, so you see many of them in the programs in this book. Not only do they help you build strength in that end position but they allow you to build awareness of what muscles should be firing and help you build more stability in your joints as you eventually move through the full range of motion.

## Eccentric

Eccentric contractions are when your muscles lengthen while actively producing force. This contraction is commonly referred to as the "lowering phase" or a "negative" because it is typically the portion of the movement when you are lowering the load , as in a squat, biceps curl, chin-up, or push-up. This is the stage of a movement that you often see programmed at a slower or longer tempo. It is often referred to as "eccentric training." Like an isometric contraction, a slow tempo will help you build stability as you gain awareness about what muscles should be firing in the movement. The eccentric portion of the movement is typically where we are the strongest and can hold more load, but this does not necessarily mean it will be easy. This is often where you'll find a lot of your soreness after a workout because of the significant demands on your muscles, but when done safely, eccentric training is one of the most effective methods to strengthen your muscles.

## Concentric

The concentric part of an exercise is when a muscle shortens while producing force—the opposite of the eccentric. I like to think of it as overcoming gravity, as in the "push" portion of a push-up, when you stand up from a squat, when you bring your dumbbells up to your shoulders in a biceps curl, or when you return to your starting position from a lunge. While focusing solely on the eccentric can result in major strength gains, training the concentric has its own strength and power benefits. You may even see some lifters drop the bar at the top of a deadlift to avoid controlling the bar in the eccentric, because they are solely focusing on the concentric, managing their fatigue. There are other ways you can steer clear of the eccentric and concentrate on the concentric, like doing a push-up from the ground and then resetting from your knees back to the ground. Doing a movement like this with the focus on the eccentric phase will help you get stronger in the full range of motion, but doing the concentric phase on its own can also help you activate different muscles.

## DECIPHERING STRENGTH JARGON

The following is terminology that you hear in the strength training world, along with a brief explanation of how each one relates to the programs in part III of this book.

### Personal Record (PR)

You'll hear a lot of people say, "I hit a PR today!" and that's a good thing! This means they may have lifted a heavier weight than their last workout for the same amount of reps, or maybe they were able to move the same weight for more reps. If you're starting from scratch and have never lifted weights before, then everything will be a PR!

### Progressive Overload

Progressive overload happens when you gradually increase the weight and repetitions for each exercise as you move through a program, but not necessarily at the same time. This is what you see in the programs in this book. As you build strength, exercises will start to feel easier with the weight you choose and repetitions prescribed. Progressive overload will help you continue to build muscle strength and avoid plateaus. This may be reflected by increasing the weight in your goblet squat from 30 pounds (13.60 kg) for 10 repetitions to 35 pounds (15.87 kg) for only 6 to 8 repetitions. You can also keep the same weight but complete more repetitions. We'll explore more about increasing weight in the next chapter.

### Load, Reps, and Sets

"Load" refers to the amount of weight you use. This could be your body weight, the weight of a dumbbell, or the amount of weight on your barbell. "Reps" is short for repetitions and refers to each individual exercise—for instance, 8 reps of a biceps curl. Sets are the number of times you will do each block of exercises, such as "2 sets of 8 reps." While the repetitions and sets will be noted in the programs, the load will not be prescribed; that will be up to you to keep track of so that you can implement your progressive overload.

## Interval

Intervals are the amount of time that you are actively working and then resting, usually with the emphasis on the work period. You may hear someone say "Do 3 sets of 20-second speed squat intervals. You'll have 40 seconds to rest in between." You would do 20 seconds of speed squats, rest for 40 seconds, do 20 seconds of speed squats again, rest for 40 again, then finish up with your third set of 20-second speed squats and be done with this exercise. This can also be referenced as "20 seconds on, 40 seconds off." Intervals are usually used for metabolic conditioning, circuit training, or as a challenge to finish a workout. Metabolic conditioning, also popularly known as *metcon*, can be an exercise that challenges you by increasing your heart rate for a short period of time to improve the efficiency of your energy systems.

## Tempo

Tempo is the rate of speed at which you move through the eccentric, end-range isometric, and concentric contractions of each movement. In this book, they are written in the order of the movement and in seconds. For example, if you have a goblet squat noted with (3, 1, 1), that means you will lower down into your squat for 3 seconds, hold it at the bottom for 1 second, and then return to your starting position for 1 second. Or if you have a dumbbell bent over row noted with (1, 3, 3), that means you will lift or pull the dumbbells up for 1 second, hold at the top for 3 seconds, and then lower the dumbbells back down for 3 seconds. If you see an "X" in place of a number, it means you won't spend a lot of time in that contraction, which implies an emphasis on power or speed. If there is no tempo noted, you will be moving at a regular tempo of (1, 1, 1), a tempo is not required (like a walking exercise), or it is a timed exercise that requires a hold. Do your best to stick to the tempos prescribed.

## Superset

A superset is when you do two exercises back-to-back with a rest before repeating it. Typically, it works different muscle groups or patterns alternately, so it could be a lower-body movement paired with an upper-body one or a pair of upper-body exercises alternating the movement pattern: one push and one pull. When you pair exercises like this, you can maximize your effort without overfatiguing the muscles.

## Circuit

Circuits are a block of three or more exercises done one after the other with short recoveries in between, and you may see them as a mix of strength, cardio, and metabolic conditioning movements. These may be broken down into repetitions or timed intervals. A lot of popular group fitness classes are taught circuit style, with a few different stations that you rotate through.

Now that you're familiar with basic anatomy, strength jargon, and equipment, let's look at what you need to get started.

# 4

# GETTING STARTED

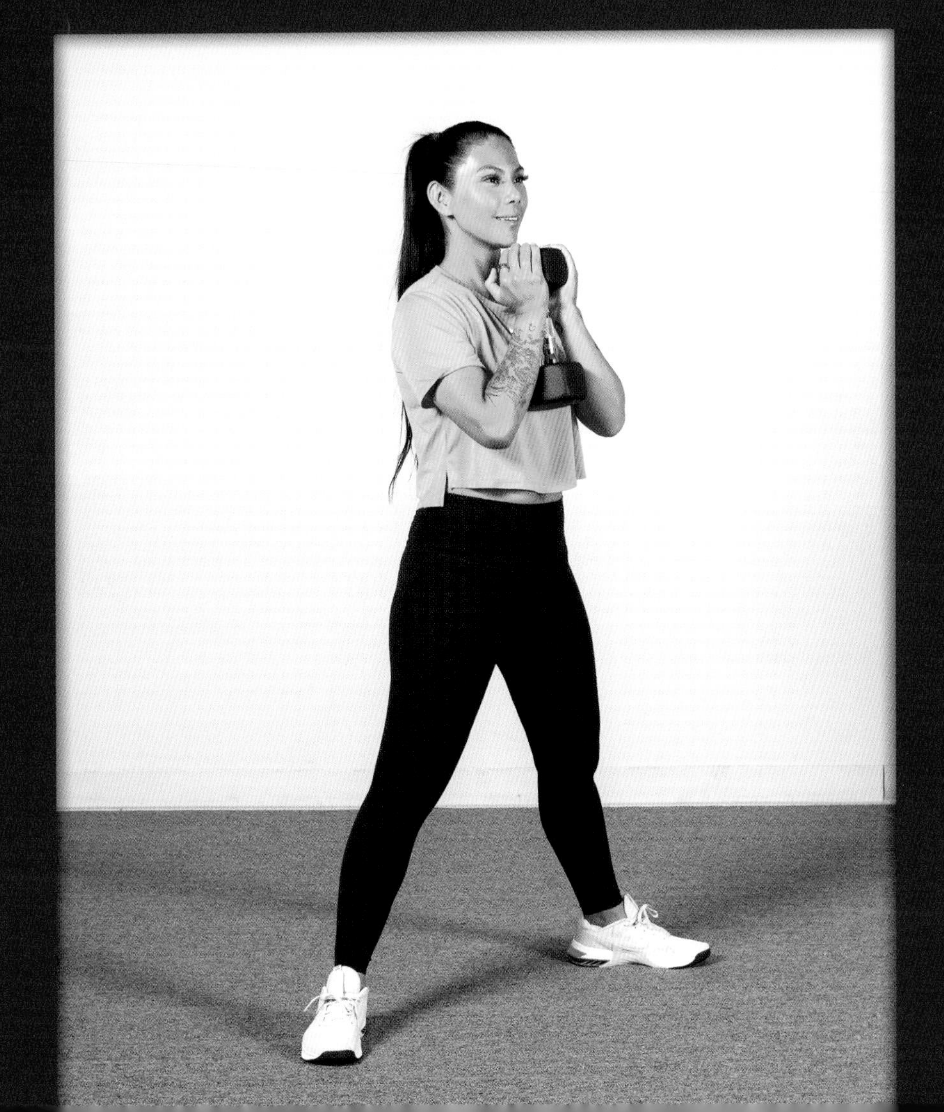

There are a lot of things to consider before getting started on any of the four programs in this book, from what you wear to what weights to pick, even which program to start with. Before getting started, be sure to check with your health care provider about whether this type of exercise is right for you at this time.

## PERFORMANCE APPAREL

Let's talk about a few different things that are important when choosing what to wear. It's important for you to wear something that will help you move freely during your workouts, but I'd also like to consider how you want to present yourself if you are working out in a public space, especially if this is a new experience for you. You should definitely wear something that you are comfortable in. Comfort is relative, though! You may feel comfortable and confident wearing short shorts and a sports bra, and that is great. You may feel comfortable wearing baggy sweatpants and an oversized tee, and that's fine too. What I'm going to dig into here is specific to your movement in strength training and the breathability of the material.

When you are working out, chances are you'll be sweating, and you'll be moving through many different ranges of motion. There are a lot of athletic wear brands out there that are associated with working out or running, and you may automatically assume they're good for that. Those brands often will have a "lifestyle" line that is meant more for a sporty look but not necessarily for performance. Imagine the free cotton tee that you may get out of a T-shirt cannon at a baseball game. Cotton does not wick away sweat. Instead it will absorb the sweat and moisture and leave you with an uncomfortable, soggy feeling. To avoid this, look for clothing that is labeled "breathable" or "wicking." Find a top that allows you to easily move your arms overhead, and if you're uncomfortable with your stomach showing, make sure it is long enough to cover it.

Keep in mind that you'll be squatting, lunging, and bridging, so the leggings or shorts you wear should be thick enough to not be see-through when stretched. Also, some tights marketed for running have zippers on the back and that can be uncomfortable when doing anything in a supine position.

Lastly, a sports bra! For women who like more support, this can be one of the most difficult things to find. Some brands have specialists who can help you with sizing and fitting, so don't be afraid to ask at a specialty store. When you find a kind you like, make sure you get at least two! It's not fun when you have to put on your smelly bra from the day before because you don't have a clean one. I recommend having your workout clothes ready for action in your gym bag or laid out the night before. Don't forget an additional bag to put your sweaty clothes in after you're done with your workout!

## FOOTWEAR

Now let's talk about what you put on your feet. You may have seen people work out barefoot, and I do advocate for this, as long as you are in a safe environment to do so and the facility allows it. Barefoot training allows your feet a higher level of proprioception, or awareness of their position in space. This can help with balance, mobility, and strength, especially in strength training.

However, training with shoes and socks is not a bad thing. You just need to have the right kind of both. For strength training, what you want to consider in socks is similar to what's important in your clothing: you want them to be comfortable and breathable. If ankle socks are your thing, make sure they don't slip down and cause a distraction during your workout. The ideal shoe for training will allow your foot to flex or point, to feel supported as you move side to side, forward and back, and help you feel grounded into the floor and maintain contact as you move weight.

I don't recommend doing strength training with shoes that are marketed toward long-distance running. Those shoes are meant to support your feet while running for a long period of time, and they typically have a lot cushioning in the forefoot and heel to help absorb shock. When you are doing a weighted movement like a squat, it is important to feel grounded in the position. A heavily cushioned running shoe may do the opposite. Let's say you're doing a single-leg Romanian deadlift for which you stand on one foot. In this particular exercise, you hinge at your hips, bringing your chest forward and toward the ground with or without a weight, all while standing on one foot. Too much cushioning in your shoe may destabilize you and possibly knock you off balance.

The bottom line in a training shoe is one that makes you feel supported while you move in different planes and for balance and weight shifts. This can mean many different things to many people and different feet, so I suggest starting with a shoe that is marketed for "training" versus running, and trying a few movements in them, like a reverse lunge or a squat.

## SELF-ASSESSMENT: BODY COMPOSITION

When it comes to assessing fitness, I am a big advocate of looking beyond that bathroom scale. The scale is a good general guide, but there are many things to keep in mind. As you go through a strength program, you build muscle, which is more dense than fat. If you are weighing yourself every day, you might not even see a change in the number, though there very well could be many changes happening in your body. Plus, weight fluctuates throughout the day, so if you choose to weigh yourself, the best time is first thing in the morning, after relieving yourself and before eating or drinking. Consistency of the variables is important when tracking your weight.

There are also a few different machines that you may find in fitness facilities or specialty clinics that assess weight along with body fat, like an InBody Scale (see figure 4.1), which measures body composition through a method called bioelectrical impedance analysis. This is a noninvasive technique using a weak electric current that flows through the body and measures voltage to calculate impedance (resistance). Typically, the measurement is done via two handles on which you rest your hands. As with a scale, it's important to keep in mind the time of day and consider what you have eaten or drunk at the time of measurement. This is a good way to get a more detailed benchmark of your body composition, but there are many other ways if you can't find access to one. I detail a few more in the next section.

An easy way to see the changes happening is to take a photo at the beginning of your fitness journey and continue to take progress photos along the way—for example, about every 2 to 3 weeks. Wear a bathing suit and take photos of your front, side, and back. I recommend setting up the camera on a tripod so it's always at the same height and take each photo in the same spot, at the same time of day, and with the same lighting. Remember, consistency is key!

You can also assess your body with a flexible tape measure. You may need someone to help you, but it is possible to do most of it on your own. Wear appropriate clothing when you measure, avoiding anything too baggy. You measure the circumference of the widest or thickest part of your upper arms, chest, thighs and hips, and you take two measurements for your waist (see figure 4.2):

- *Upper arm:* Measure around the thickest part of your arm, typically around your biceps.
- *Chest:* Measure around the widest part of your chest, typically around your nipple line.
- *Hips:* Measure around the widest part of your hips, typically just above your crotch.
- *Upper thigh:* Measure around the thickest part of your thigh, about halfway between your knee and hip.
- *Calf:* Measure around the thickest part of your calf, usually about 1/4 of the way down from your knee.
- *Lower waist and natural waist:* Measure right above your belly button and also right below your belly button

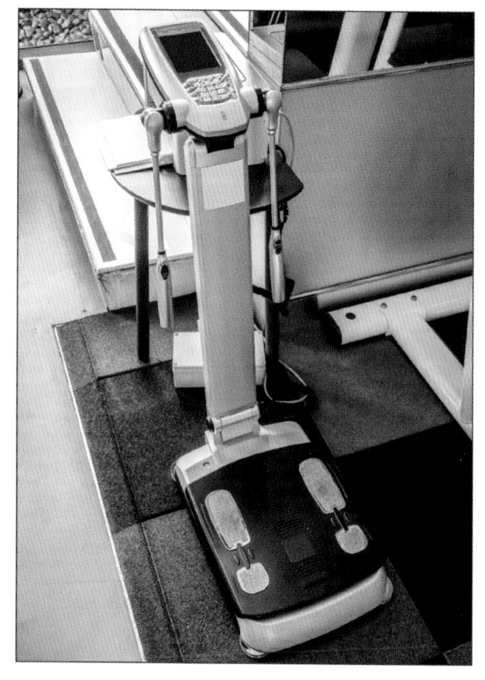

**FIGURE 4.1** A bioelectrical impedance machine (BIA) can be used to track body composition.
Vudhikul Ocharoen/iStockphoto/Getty Images

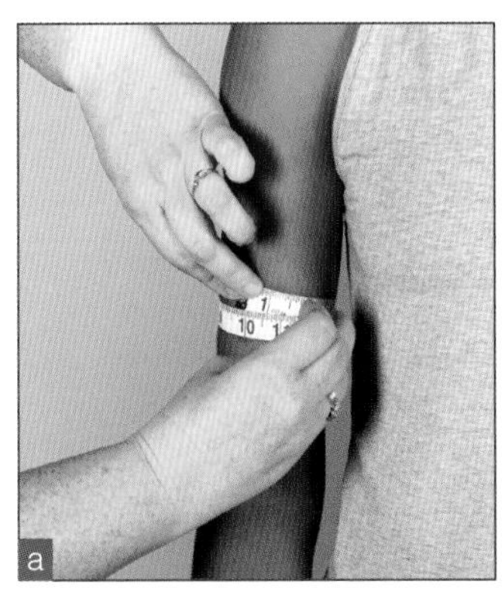


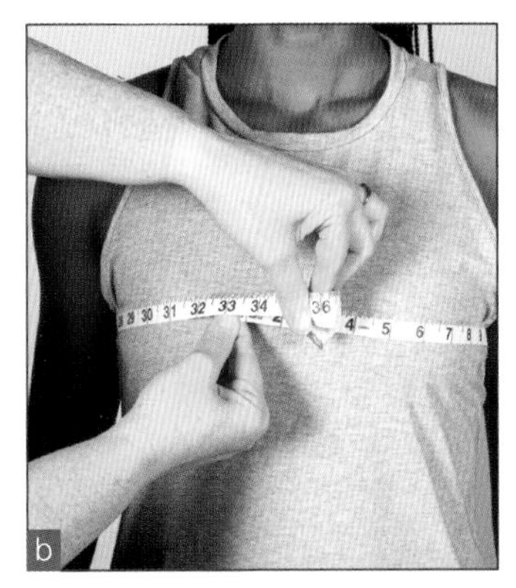


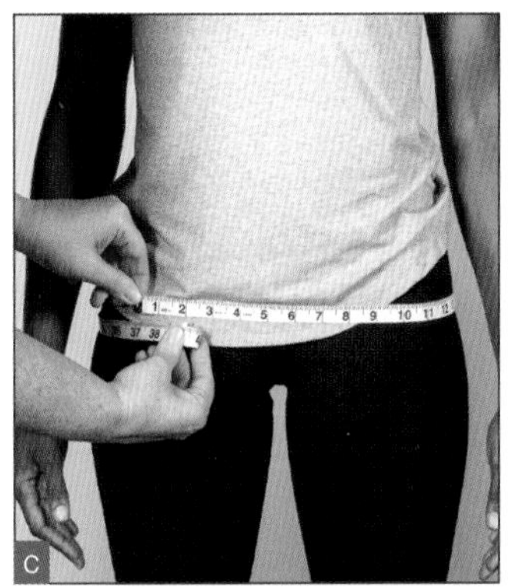


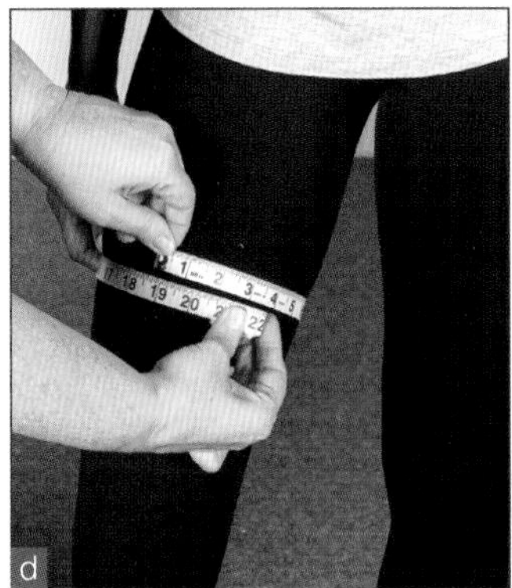


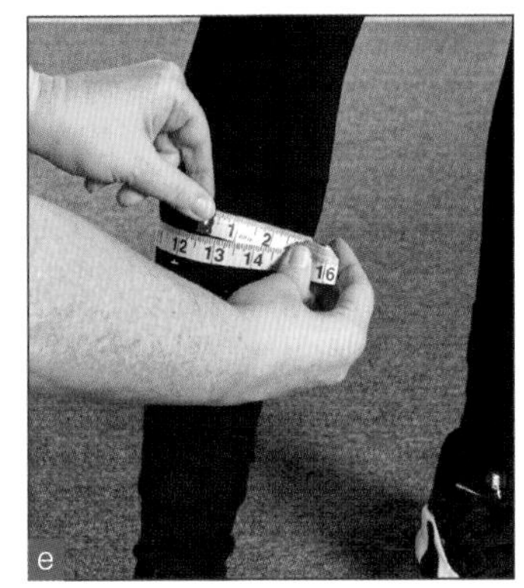


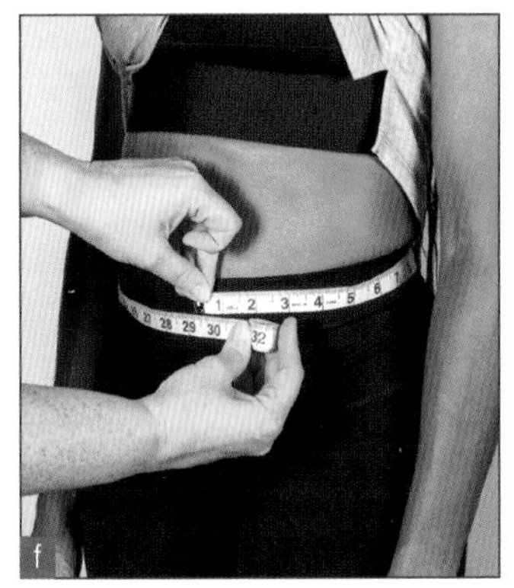


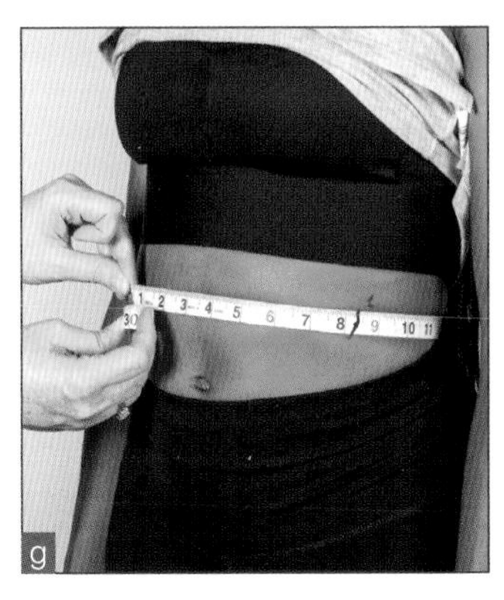


**FIGURE 4.2** Use these model examples as a guide to measure each of the following body parts: (*a*) upper arm, (*b*) chest, (*c*) hips, (*d*) upper thigh, (*e*) calf, (*f*) lower waist, and (*g*) natural waist.

As with the photos, a good frequency for measuring would be every 2 to 3 weeks, and keeping constant variables.

## SELF-ASSESSMENT: SKILLS

I mentioned that I am a big advocate for looking beyond the scale, and that is where assessing your skill comes in. This could be as simple as performing your first push-up on your toes or doing your first pull-up, or you can get as detailed as using a specific weight for your deadlift or bench press. As a strength coach, watching improvement happen is what I live for, and I've found that a lot of people's general goals of weight loss and toned muscle naturally follow when they focus on achieving a skill or a certain personal record.

There are many ways you can assess your skill level, but what follows is a basic skills test that you can use to help you. You may need to preview the exercises in the following chapters in order to execute them if you are unsure of them (page numbers for where they appear in this book follow each exercise). Keep in mind that this skills test is a workout in itself, so be sure to warm up adequately! It will be challenging, but the beauty of it is in seeing how you progress with these movements over the span of your training. I recommend keeping track of your progress by recording the date, your measurements, and other training details, and revisiting the skills test every 4 weeks.

## Grip Strength

In all three of these movements, you should hold for as long as you can without losing form. I have indicated what weight to use. If you are unable to use that weight, pick a weight that's neither too easy nor too difficult and record that weight. Mark the time when you have to let go of the bar or lower the weight. If you are able to hold for the maximum (max) time, mark that down and give yourself the option of picking a heavier weight for the exercises that indicate that as a choice.

Dead hang: total hold time (max 90 sec); page 48

Farmer carry (35 lb [15.87 kg] each hand): total hold time (max 90 sec); page 43

Front rack (20 lb [9.07 kg] each hand): total hold time (max 90 sec); page 45

## Core Strength

In these five exercises, you will focus not only on your abs but also on your hips and glutes. These exercises are all body-weight holds, so there is no option to add any weight. If you are able to complete all exercises with the max hold, record how the exercises feel to you on a scale of 1 to 10, with 10 being the most difficult.

Hollow hold: total hold time (max 90 sec); page 60

High plank: total hold time (max 90 sec); page 58

Side plank: total hold time (max 90 sec each side); page 56

Single-leg bridge: total hold time (max 90 sec each side); variation of bridge found on page 82

Copenhagen 90/90: total hold time (max 45 sec each side); page 61

## General Strength

In these exercises, you test your maximum number of reps with the weight I suggest. If you can't move the weight or you are completing the max number of reps easily, change the weight and make sure to record what you are using to keep track of your benchmark. If you are unable to complete some of the body-weight movements, that's OK! Mark it as "none yet," and be motivated to get stronger!

Chin-up (assisted or unassisted) (underhand/supinated grip): total number of reps (max 15); page 128 or 127

Dumbbell bridge (35 lb [15.87 kg]): total number of reps (max 15); page 81

Push-up on bench: total number of reps (max 20). Place your hands on a bench or box and make a note of the height of the bench or box to keep track. The higher the box or bench, the less challenging it will be; page 99

Goblet squat (20 lb [9.07 kg]): total number of reps (max 20); page 66

Dumbbell overhead press (10 lb [4.53 kg]): total number of reps (max 15); page 108

Dumbbell Romanian deadlift (15 lb [6.80 kg] in each hand): total number of reps (max 15); page 85

Inverted row (overhand/pronated grip; indicate if knees are bent or legs straight): total number of reps (max 15); page 117

Goblet stationary lunge or split squat (variation of dumbbell stationary lunge or split squat; 10 lb [4.53 kg]): total number of reps each side (max 15 each side); page 75

Body-weight single-leg Romanian deadlift: total number of reps on each side without falling over or losing balance (max 10 each side); dumbbell single-leg Romanian deadlift found on page 87

Getting through this basic skills test will not only start you off with a good assessment of your baseline strength—it can also help you figure out what weights to use when it's time to start the programs. In chapter 10, Create Your Optimal Program, I go into detail of how to determine load (weight) for your workouts.

# GOAL SETTING

Setting a goal for fitness and wellness is important, but it's even more imperative that you set specific, achievable goals. Here's a helpful framework called SMART goals.

**S:** Specific

**M:** Measurable

**A:** Achievable

**R:** Realistic

**T:** Timely

SMART goals have been my own guide for both my fitness and my business! It's so easy to say, "I want to get in shape" or "I want to lose weight," but what's missing from both of these statements? Answer: the time range, specificity, and a way to measure if you've reached your goal. A perfect time to set your training goals is after you've completed your self-assessment and skills tests. This will help you to make realistic, specific, and achievable goals.

In the following sections are some examples of SMART goals.

## Ava

Ava, 25, has never worked out on her own before, but she played soccer in high school. She knows she wants to get a good routine going, so she picked up this book. During her skills assessment, she was able to hang from the bar for 5 seconds but couldn't do any pull-ups or chin ups during her skills test. (Pull-ups differ from chin-ups in that pull-ups use a pronated grip and chin-ups use a supinated grip. See chapter 5 for more on this.)

### Ava's SMART Goals

"I will start a strength program and work out 3 days a week for 3 months."

"I will be able to perform 3 pull-ups at the end of the 3 months and be able to hang from the bar for at least 15 seconds"

Ava's goals are realistic in that they are measurable—they're expressed in concrete terms within a specific time span. Because her initial skills test showed that she couldn't hang from the pull-up bar for more than 5 seconds and she couldn't do pull-ups, she is focused on gaining enough strength to hold onto the bar for a little bit longer than she was previously able and to do 3 pull-ups. This gives her a realistic goal of adding at least 1 pull-up and 5 seconds each month. That is definitely achievable!

## Cameron

Cameron, 32, has had a consistent workout routine for many years, but she wants to get more targeted in her training. After her skills test, she realizes she has very strong legs and can complete the max reps for her lower body, but can complete only 5 push-ups on the bench.

**Cameron's SMART Goals**

"I will do strength training 3 times a week and be able to complete 10 push-ups on the bench after the first month of my program."

"By the end of my 12-week program, I will complete 5 push-ups on the floor!"

Because Cameron already has a consistent workout routine, she is more specific in her goal. With her good foundation of strength, she wants to develop a stronger upper body. Her goal to complete a realistic number of push-ups by the end of her first month is timely, and she knows she can progress to performing those 5 push-ups on the floor by the end of the program.

## Yvette

Yvette, 42, has been on a regular workout schedule, doing spin classes and Pilates two or three times a week. She is interested in starting a strength program, but isn't sure where to begin. She did her skills test and was able to complete 5 reps of the overhead press and goblet squats, but was unable to do the stationary lunge or single-leg Romanian deadlift. She also wants to work on balance.

**Yvette's SMART Goals**

"I will focus on strength training 2 or 3 times a week, and also attend yoga once a week for 12 weeks."

"I will do 10 reps of body-weight single-leg Romanian deadlift and 10 reps of stationary lunge on each side with 10-pound dumbbells by the end of my 12-week program."

After realizing she wasn't able to do the single-leg movements very well during her skills test, Yvette wanted to achieve better balance. She knows that incorporating yoga into her routine could help her in addition to her strength training. She also gave herself an achievable number of reps to complete by the end of her 12-week program.

## Scarlett

Scarlett, 27, is serious about her strength training, making it a habit to lift weights at least 3 times a week since she was 21. She is focused on getting stronger and sculpting muscle, but she realizes she never tracks the weight that she uses when she works out, even though she has a general idea of the load. Upon completion of her assessment, she was able to complete the max for all the lower-body and upper-body movements.

**Scarlett's SMART Goals**

"I will track all the loads for the exercises in my 12-week program."

"I will hit a 225-pound hip thrust and 95-pound bench press by the end of the 12 weeks."

Scarlett is stating the specific weight she plans to use because that is something she hasn't done in the past, and this will help her track her progress. She knows that she generally lifts about 180 pounds (81.64 kg) for her hip thrust and 95pounds (43.09 kg) for her bench press, but now she is going to hold herself accountable by tracking the weight and setting a realistic goal to achieve.

In all of these goals, you'll notice the focus is on skills and accountability. I've found my clients experience more success when they pinpoint these things rather than obsess over the number on a scale. In fact, I've had some clients who were so focused on these skills and accountability goals that they even forgot to weigh and measure themselves until I reminded them! Keep in mind that I am not discouraging you from setting a goal focused on weight, but I love the mindset that comes with accountability. It's OK if you aren't sure of your specific goal just yet. I encourage you to write down some ideas, explore the rest of this book and review the programs, then get more detailed with your goals, keeping SMART in mind.

# PART II

# LEARNING THE EXERCISES

# 5

# CARRY, GRIP, AND ANTIMOVEMENT

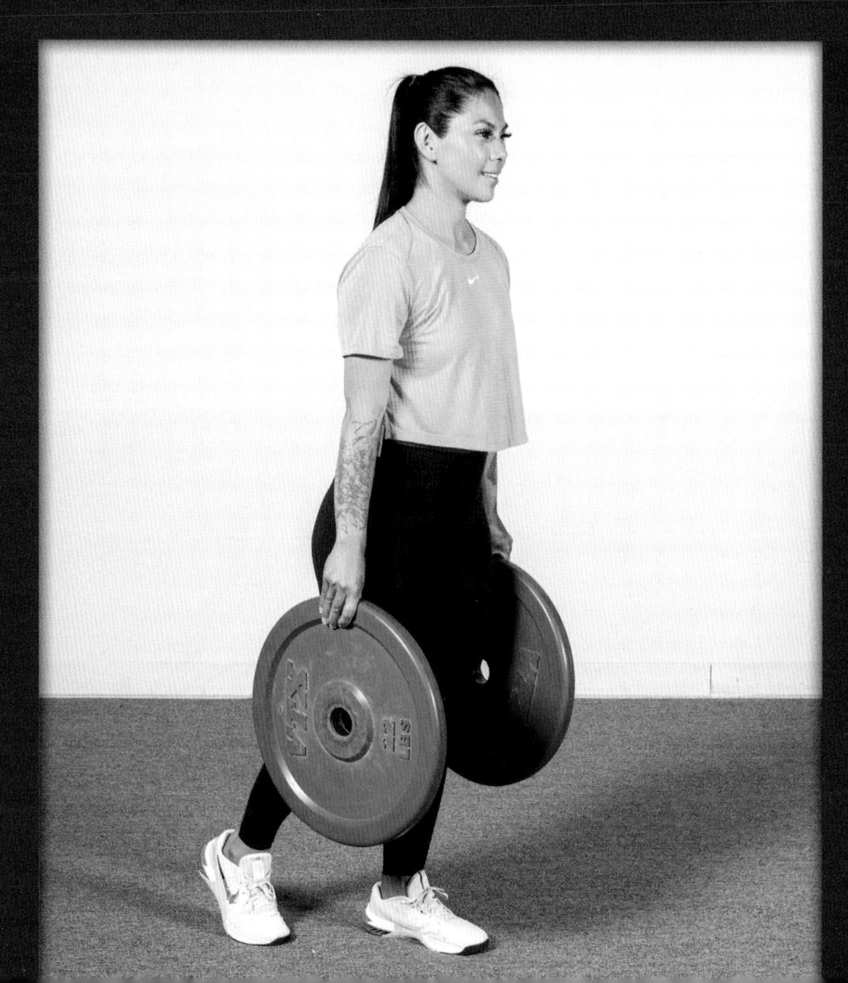

The carry and grip exercises in this chapter are vital foundational exercises for strength. They work the flexors of your forearm. Strengthening your forearms helps improve your strength for the many tasks you perform in a day, like carrying groceries or opening a pickle jar. It's likely you'll be lifting heavier weights as you progress through the programs in this book, so you'll need to make sure that you can hold that weight. The stronger your grip, the more weight you can handle and the more repetitions you can do. When adding movement while gripping, stabilization of your joints adds a whole new level of challenge to your muscles, and that's where carry exercises come in. *Note*: For any of the carry movements, if you don't have the space to walk, you can march in place for the desired number of steps.

## MARCHING IN PLACE

If you do not have the space to walk for a carry exercise, you can march in place, counting the amount of desired steps *(a-b)*.

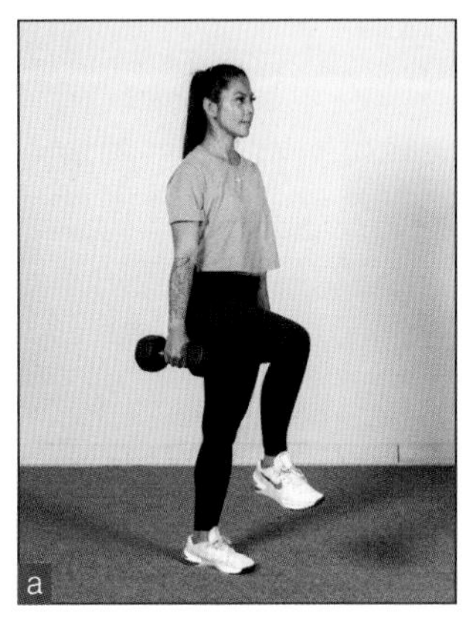
a

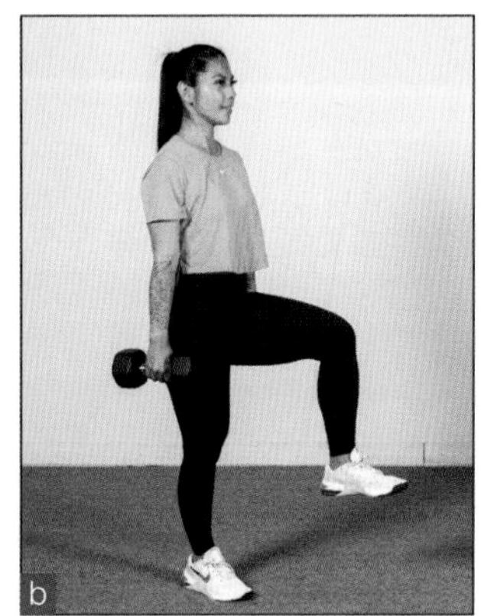
b

"Antimovement" is a general name for the core stability exercises in this chapter that include antirotation or antiflexion. It may seem confusing, but "anti" here doesn't mean rotational and flexion movements are bad! You should be rotating and moving your spine, but these movements help strengthen and protect your lower back, shoulders, hips, and spine while you rotate and hold external load, or weight. This can support you in everyday movement, like putting on a seat belt, holding a child, lifting a heavy box from the ground, or swinging a tennis racket. The antimovement exercises featured in this chapter are great as a warm-up to help activate your core and prepare you for lifting weight. They are also added onto some of the strength circuits or supersets to challenge your core under fatigue.

## FARMER CARRY

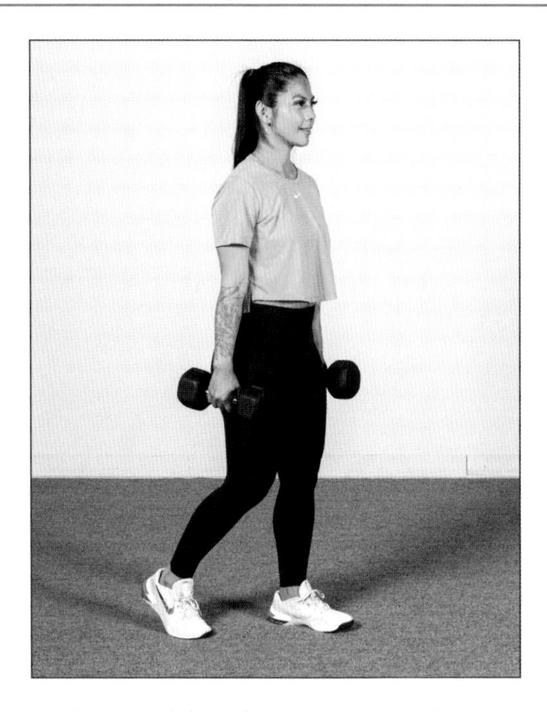

1. Stand with a weight in each hand, arms at your sides, and palms facing each other while bracing your core.
2. Keep the weights at your side as you walk forward slowly, keeping your chest open and posture tall.
3. As you walk, keep your weight evenly distributed so that you are not shifting your weight drastically from one side to another.
4. Upon completion of reps or distance, slowly lower your weight back to the floor or rack with control.

### Things to Keep in Mind

- Keep your shoulders stacked over your rib cage and rib cage stacked over hips, with your pelvis tucked.
- Do not put one foot directly in front of the other as though you were on a tightrope.
- Do not "waddle" side to side with the weight.

## SUITCASE CARRY

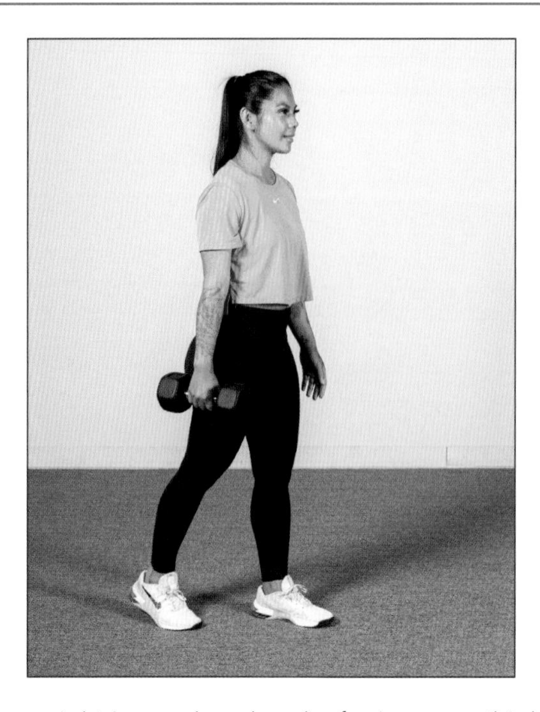

1. Stand with a weight in one hand, palm facing your thighs, while bracing your core.
2. Keep the weight at your side as you walk forward slowly, keeping your chest open and posture tall.
3. Upon completion of reps or distance, slowly lower your weight to the floor or rack with control.
4. Repeat on the other side.

### Things to Keep in Mind

- Keep your shoulders stacked over your rib cage and rib cage stacked over hips, with your pelvis tucked.
- Use your core to keep your shoulders, ribs, and hips stacked as you walk, making sure your weight is not shifted over to one side.
- Do not walk like you are on a tightrope.

# RACK CARRY

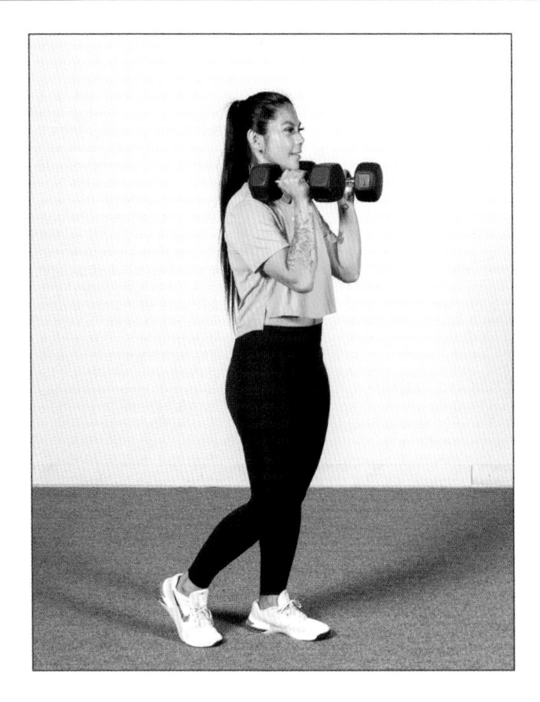

1. Stand with a dumbbell in each hand, arms at your sides, and palms facing each other while bracing your core.
2. Lift the dumbbells up to shoulder height, palms facing each other, keeping your elbows close to your rib cage. (This is known as "rack position.")
3. Keep the weights in the rack position as you slowly walk forward, making sure you are not leaning back and that your chest is open and posture is tall.
4. Upon completion of reps or distance, slowly lower your weights back down with control.

## KETTLEBELL RACK POSITION

### Things to Keep in Mind

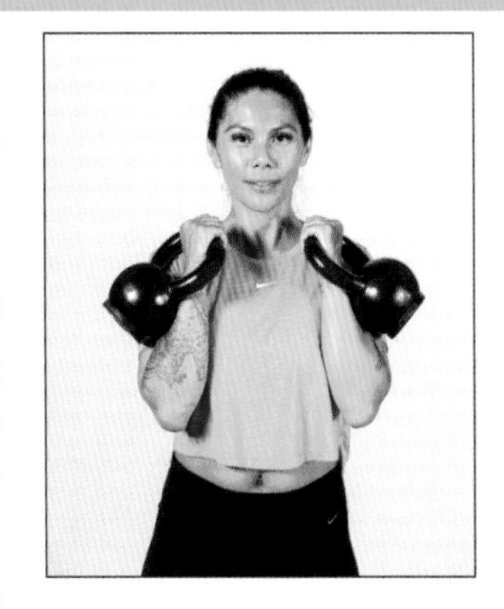

- Keep your wrists straight, not bent forward or back.
- This is an advanced position.
- As the weight gets heavier, the back of your wrist will take some adjustment. It may be tender at first, but it may become less sore over time as you lift more frequently.
- Be mindful of wearable devices, watches, or jewelry, as the kettlebells can damage them.

# HIGH GOBLET CARRY

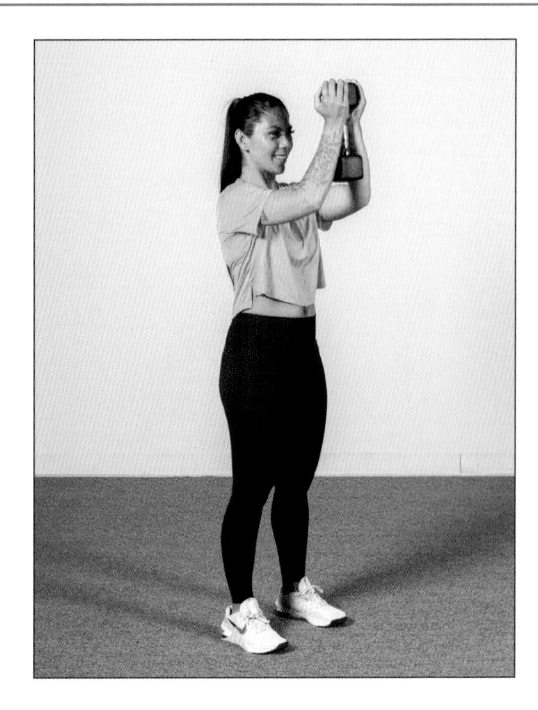

1. Hold a dumbbell vertically, with both hands, in front of your chest.
2. Lift the dumbbell with both hands so it is line with your forehead and your elbows are in line with your shoulders.
3. Keep your rib cage stacked as you hold the dumbbell in this high position and slowly walk forward.
4. Upon competition of reps or distance, slowly lower your weight back down with control.

## Things to Keep in Mind

- If your mobility does not allow you to keep your elbows up high and you feel like you are puffing your chest out, then lower the dumbbell a little bit.
- Do not walk like you are on a tightrope.

# PLATE PINCH HOLD

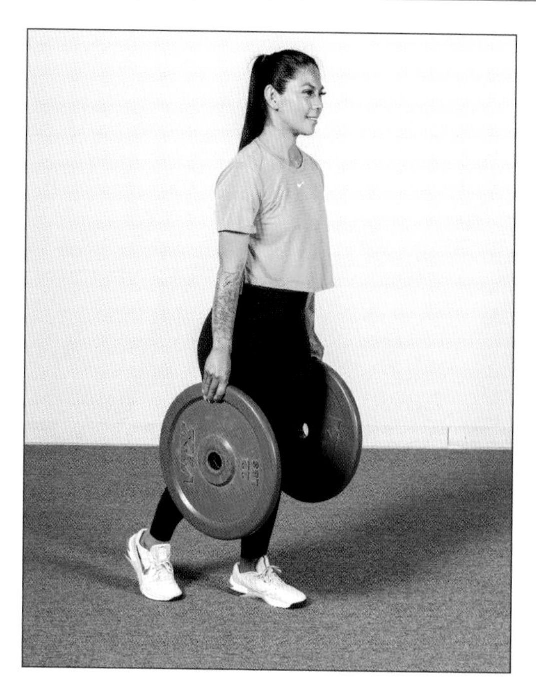

1. Stand with two weight plates on the ground, one on each side of your feet.
2. Pinch each plate with your fingertips so that your thumbs are one side and the other fingers on the other side
3. Stand up and hold the plates by your sides, with arms straight, for the desired amount of time.

## Things to Keep in Mind

- This is best done using standard size cast-iron plates without handles.

# DEAD HANG

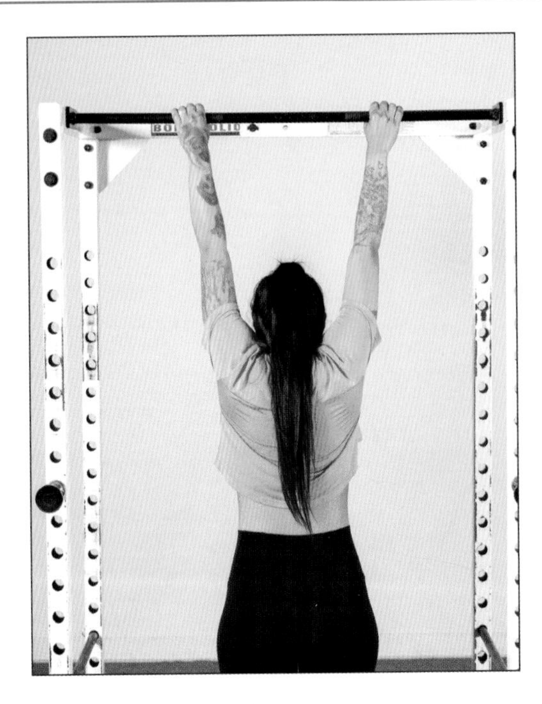

1. Stand on a sturdy bench or sturdy box that you can step on—like a plyometric box you jump onto—if needed, so that you can grab onto the pull-up bar.
2. Place your hands shoulder distance apart or slightly wider, and use an overhand closed grip on the bar.
3. Allow your body to hang from the bar so that everything but your grip is relaxed.
4. Hold for the desired amount of time.

## Things to Keep in Mind

- Make sure your hands are wrapped all the way around the bar.
- Let the rest of your body relax into the hang.

# ACTIVE HANG

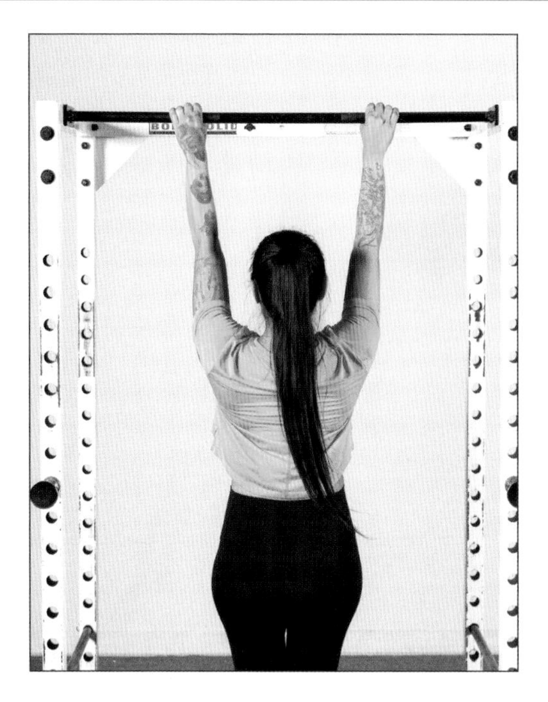

1. Stand on a sturdy bench or plyo box, if needed, so that you can grab onto the pull-up bar.
2. Place your hands shoulder distance apart or slightly wider, and use an overhand closed grip on the bar.
3. Keeping your arms straight, pull your shoulder blades down and pull your rib cage in so that you can feel your core engage.
4. Hold for the desired amount of time.

## Things to Keep in Mind

- Make sure your hands are wrapped all the way around the bar.
- Keep your whole body engaged when hanging.

# PALOFF PRESS

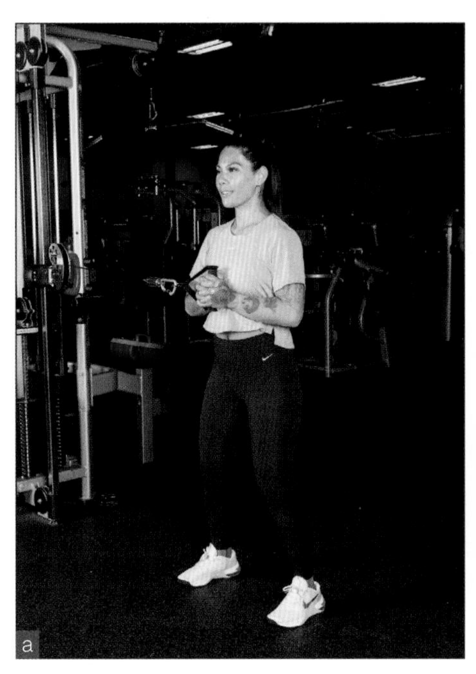
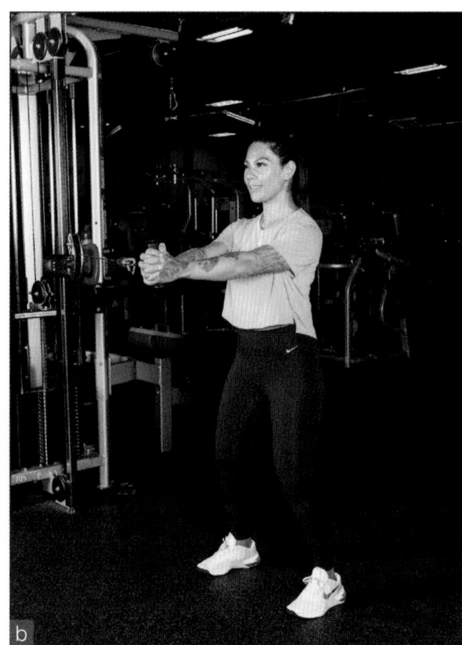

1. Adjust a cable arm or anchor a superband to a sturdy object.
2. With two hands, grab the cable handle or superband and hold it at chest level, elbows bent.
3. Orient your body to be parallel with the anchor when the cable or superband is pushed away from anchor point (one side of your body faces the anchor point) and you are standing far enough way so that there is a little tension in the cable or superband (*a*).
4. Press the cable handle or superband away from you, straightening your arms so that you can feel your core engage, keeping your shoulders away from your ears, rib cage in, and pelvis neutral (*b*).
5. Hold for 1 to 2 seconds (or desired amount of time).
6. Bend the elbows and bring the cable handle or superband back slowly to your chest. Complete the desired number of repetitions.

## Things to Keep in Mind

- Make sure you are not "biceps curling" the superband or cable to your chest, but pressing it straight out and pulling it back in.
- Keep your shoulders away from your ears by keeping your back and core muscles engaged.

## Variations

- These can be done in different stances, such as half kneeling stance (*c*) or staggered stance (*d*).

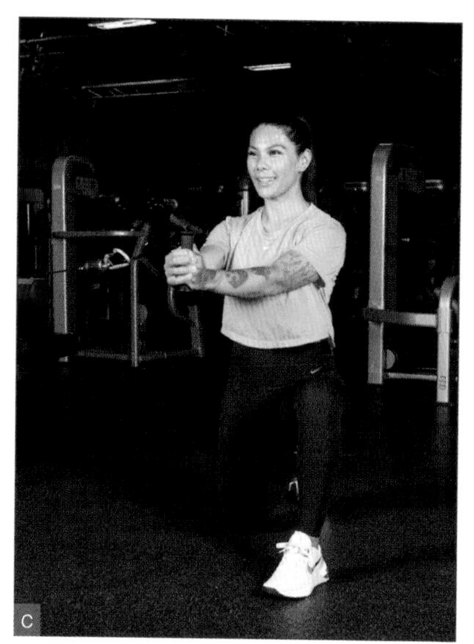
c

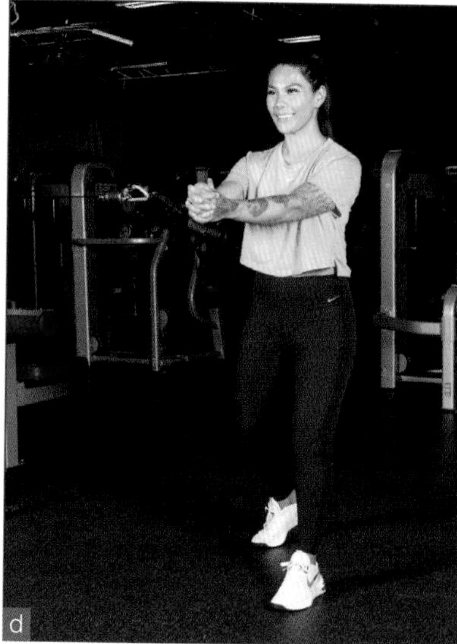
d

## BIRD DOG

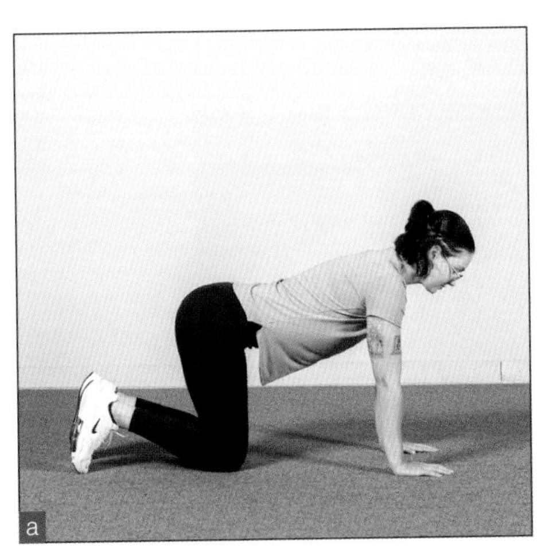


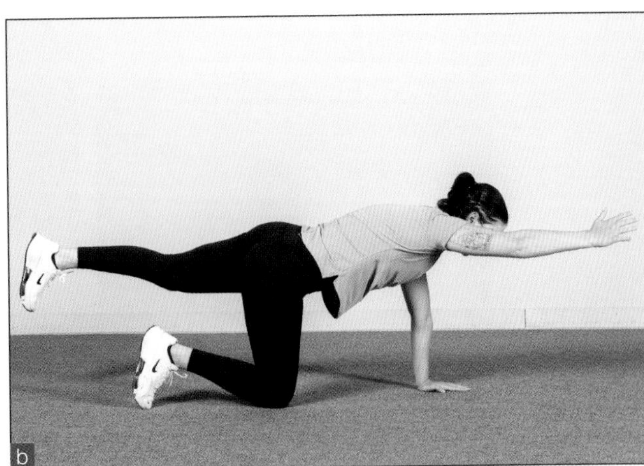


1. On your hands and knees, align your hands under your shoulders and your knees under your hips, with toes tucked under (*a*).
2. Keeping your trunk stable, extend one arm out in front of you with your pinky on the ground, while simultaneously extending the opposite leg out, straightening your knee (keep your toe on the ground).
3. To start, your toe and pinky will touch the ground. As you get stronger, the goal is to eventually raise the arm so that your biceps is near your ear and the leg extended behind you is in line with the rest of your body without letting your lower back sway (*b*).
4. Hold for 1 to 2 seconds (or desired amount of time), then return the arm and leg to the start position.
5. Repeat with the opposite arm and leg. Continue to alternate sides for the desired number of repetitions.

### Things to Keep in Mind

- Do not let your lower back arch excessively as you reach your arms and legs out.
- Focus on keeping your spine in a neutral position.

## Variation

### Bird Dog Tuck

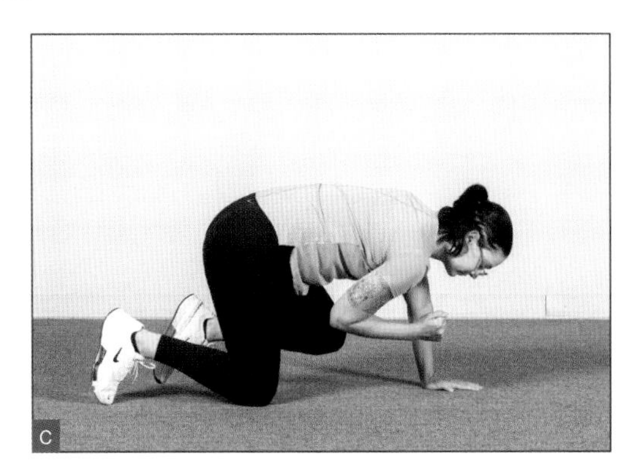


1. Still keeping your trunk stable and core engaged, when lowering the arm and leg toward the floor, bring the elbow and knee of the extended arm and leg toward each other, while rounding your back and tucking your chin (c).
2. Extend the arm and leg back out to starting position (do not alternate sides). Complete the desired number of reps.
3. Another option is to perform the motions above with the arm and the leg coming toward each other, alternating sides rather than staying on one side and then switching.

## Things to Keep in Mind

- Do not let your lower back arch excessively as you reach your arms and legs out, but as you bring your elbow and knee together, it is OK to round your back.

# DEADBUG

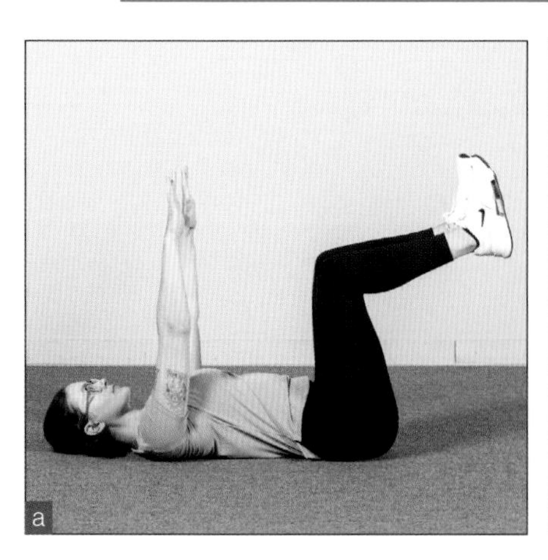

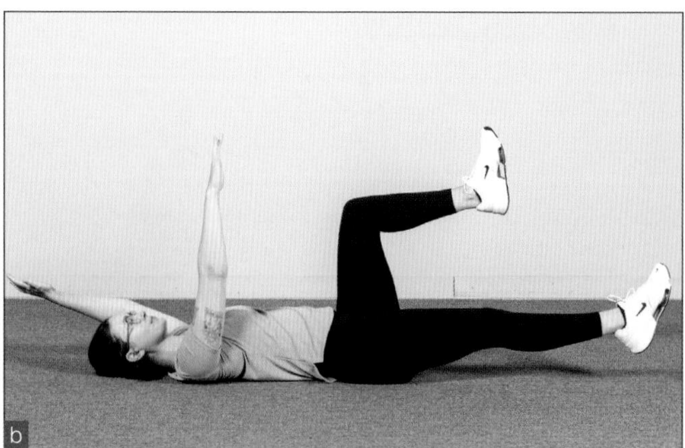

1. In a supine position (on your back), bend your knees to 90 degrees with your knees over your hips (known as "tabletop position") and feet flexed. Extend your arms from your shoulders, with your hands reaching toward the ceiling. This is your starting position (*a*).
2. Keeping one arm still extended toward the ceiling, move the other arm backward, past your head, toward the floor, so that your biceps are in line with your head. Simultaneously extend the opposite leg straight toward the floor (*b*).
3. Hold for 1 to 2 seconds (or desired amount of time), then bring the arm and leg back to the starting position.
4. Repeat on the other side. Continue to alternate for the desired number of repetitions.

## Things to Keep in Mind

- Your pelvis and rib cage should be in a neutral position.
- You do not need to have your back flat on the ground, but do not let your lower back arch excessively as you extend your arms and legs.

# SUPINE ISOMETRIC HIP FLEXION

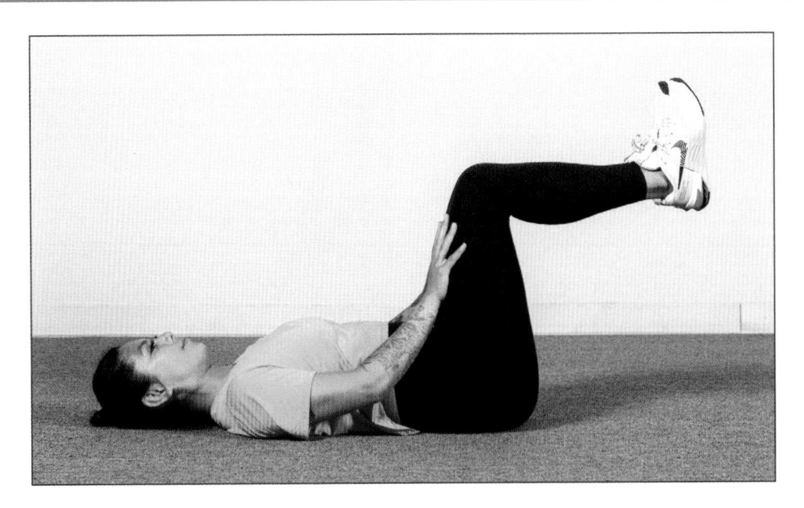

1. In a supine position (on your back), bend your knees to 90 degrees with your knees over your hips in tabletop position and feet flexed.
2. Keeping your legs in the same position, press a hand into each thigh and hold for the desired amount of time.

## Things to Keep in Mind

- Keep tension between your hands and thighs for the desired amount of time.
- Make sure your keeping tension out of your shoulders and that they aren't scrunching up.
- Take deep exhales through your mouth to use your abdominals.

# SIDE PLANK

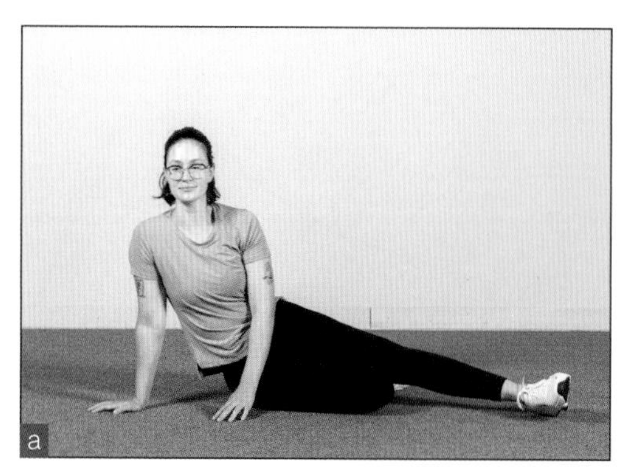


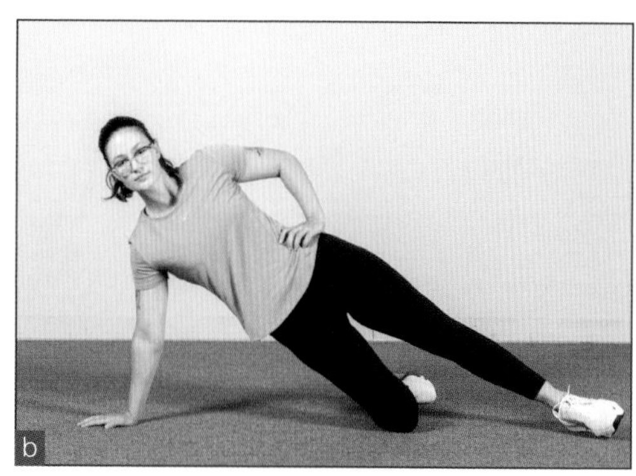


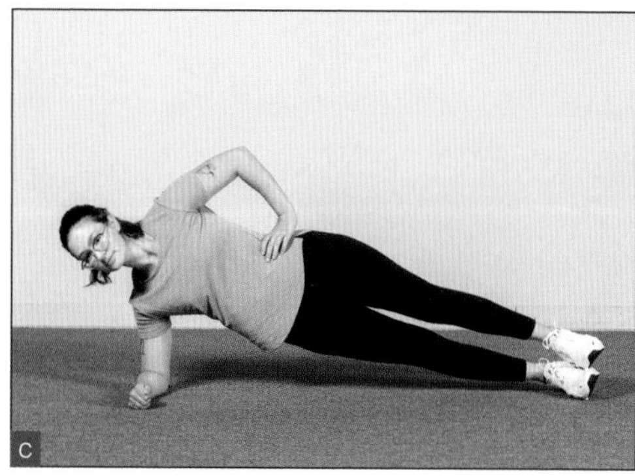


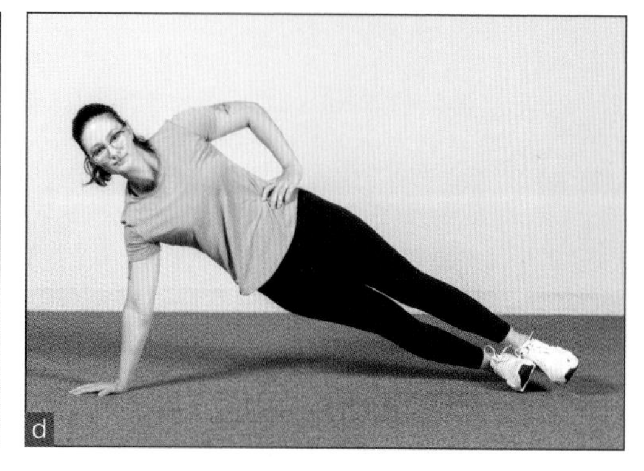


The side plank can be done on an elbow or on a hand with the arm fully extended. It will be listed in the programs in part III as "forearm side plank" or "high side plank."

1. Begin by lying on the floor on your side (*a*).
    - **High side plank:** place one hand under your shoulder and fully extend your arm so that it is supporting your body (*b*).
    - **Forearm side plank:** bend your elbow so that your forearm is on the ground with your elbow under your shoulder and hand in a fist or palm flat on the floor (*c*).
2. Lift your hips off the floor. Keep your bottom knee bent and top leg extended.
3. Stack your shoulders and hips on top of each other while keeping your rib cage in, not letting your hips sag down to the ground.
4. Hold for the desired amount of time.
5. To progress this, extend your bottom leg so that the foot of the top leg is staggered in front of the bottom foot (*d*).
6. To progress further, stack your legs on top of each other.

## Things to Keep in Mind

- Make sure you are not puffing out your chest.
- Keep your elbow or hand under your shoulder while you "press the floor away" by using your shoulders to stabilize you.

## Variation

### Side Plank Leg Lift

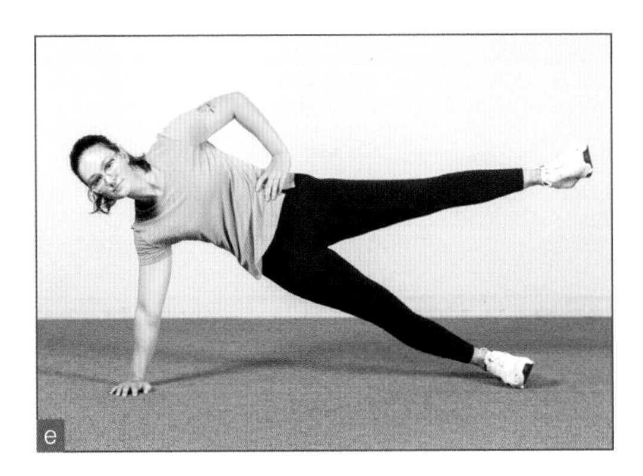


1. Set up for side plank and hold.
2. Lift your top leg up toward the ceiling and hold for 1 to 2 seconds (e).
3. Lower the leg with control and repeat for the desired amount of time or number of repetitions.
4. Repeat on the other side.

# PLANK

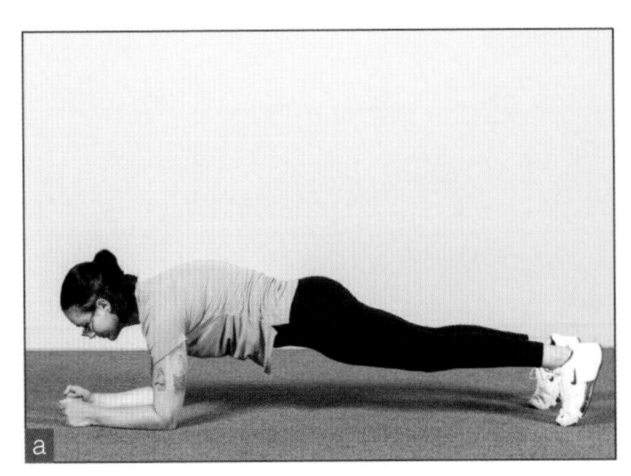


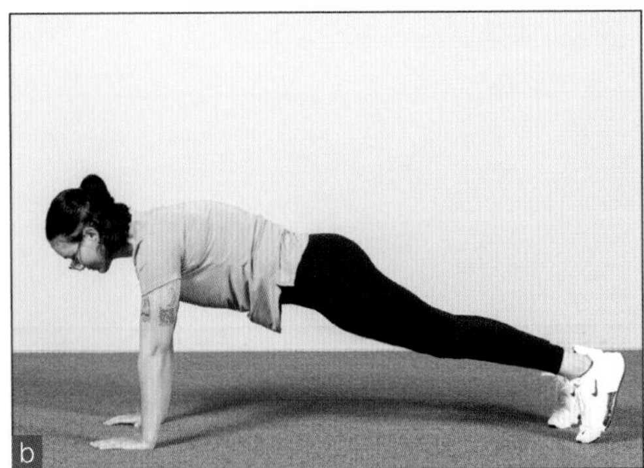


The plank can be done on elbows or on your hands with your arms fully extended. It will be listed in the programs in part III as "forearm plank" or "high plank."

1. With your feet about hip-width apart, place your hands or elbows under your shoulders and press them into the floor as you lift your body off the floor. If in high plank, the arms should be fully extended.
2. Keep your neck neutral with your gaze right between your hands if you are in forearm plank (*a*) or right past your fingertips if you are in a high plank (*b*). Engage your core by keeping your spine neutral, and keep your breathing steady.
3. Hold for the desired amount of time.

## Things to Keep in Mind

- Make sure your elbows or hands are aligned under your shoulders and you "press the floor away" by using your shoulders to stabilize you.
- Keep your rib cage in and your pelvis tucked.
- Your hips should not be up in the air or sagging.

## Variations

### Modified Plank on Knees

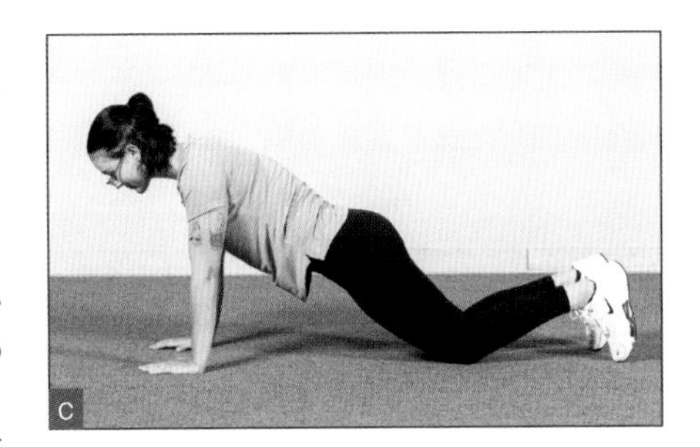


Position yourself in the plank position, but rest your weight on your knees instead of your toes (*c*).

#### Things to Keep in Mind

- Make sure hips are low and you are in a straight line, instead of a tabletop or hands-and-knees position.
- Use padding under your knees if necessary.

### Shoulder Tap

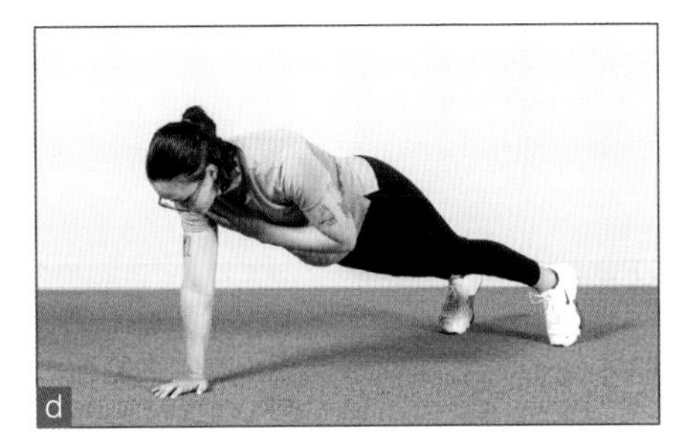


1. Set up for a plank.
2. Bring one hand toward your opposite shoulder, keeping your hips stable (*d*). Then move your hand back to the starting position and repeat with the other hand.
3. Continue to alternate sides for the desired number of repetitions.

#### Things to Keep in Mind

- The wider your feet are in this position, the more stability you have.
- To make this move easier, you can start on your knees or take your feet out wider.
- To make it more challenging, place the feet closer together.

# HOLLOW HOLD

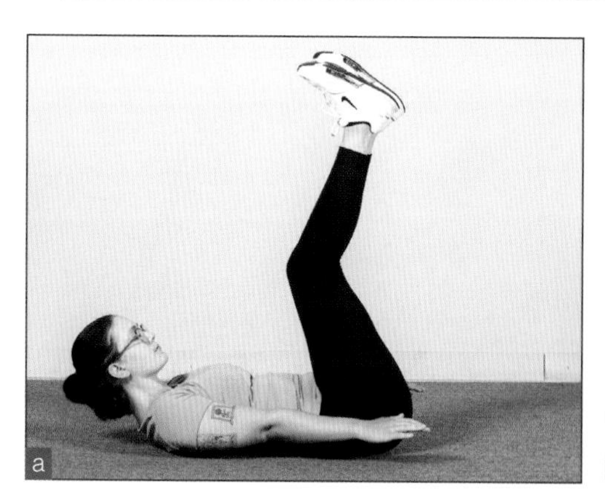
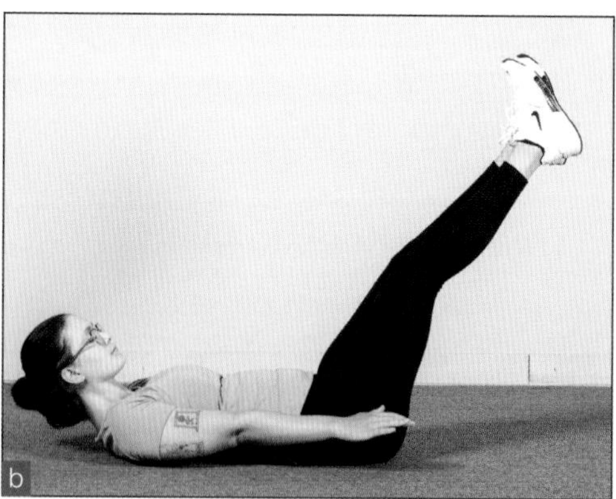

1. Lie on your back with your hands by your sides and legs off the floor; knees can be bent or legs fully extended toward the sky.
2. Lift your head and shoulders off the ground with your chin tucked, so that you are in a crunch position, then lift your arms off the ground next to you with your palms facing up toward the sky (*a*).
3. Lower your legs slowly to the lowest point where you can keep your core engaged and belly "scooped," like the letter C (*b*).
4. Hold for the desired amount of time.
5. To progress this movement, extend your arms overhead.

## Things to Keep in Mind

- Lower is not better on this exercise if your lower back comes off the ground.
- It is OK if your legs are extended straight up in the air or your knees are bent slightly.

# COPENHAGEN 90/90

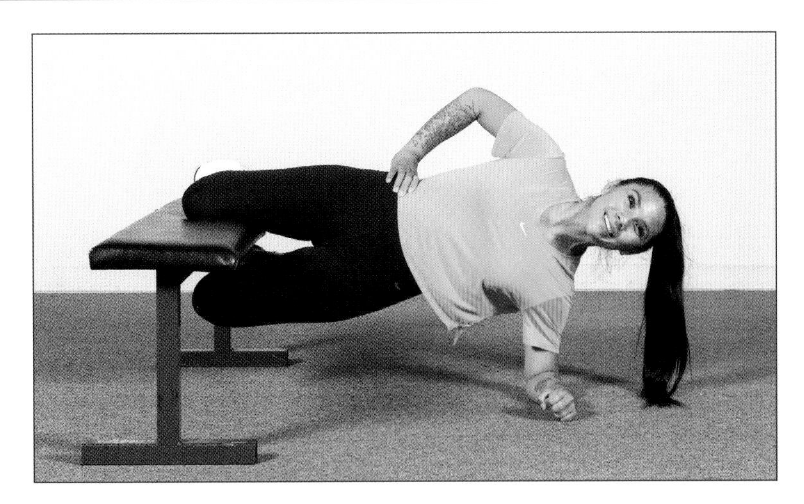

1. Use a sturdy box or bench that is about 18 inches (45.72 cm) high.
2. Lie on your side, perpendicular to the bench or box, with your feet close to the bench or box.
3. Position your bottom elbow as if you were going to perform a side plank and bend both knees.
4. Bring your top knee to the top of the box or bench. (Your calf should be parallel to the bench.) Let it support your weight, and let your other knee hang freely off the ground.
5. Support yourself with the elbow that is on the ground, keeping your pelvis tucked and your body as straight as you can.
6. Hold for the desired amount of time, then repeat on the other side.

## Things to Keep in Mind

- This is an advanced move. If the 18-inch (45.72 cm) box or bench is too high or the exercise feels extremely difficult, start with a lower box or hold the position for less time.

# 6

# KNEE DOMINANT AND HIP DOMINANT

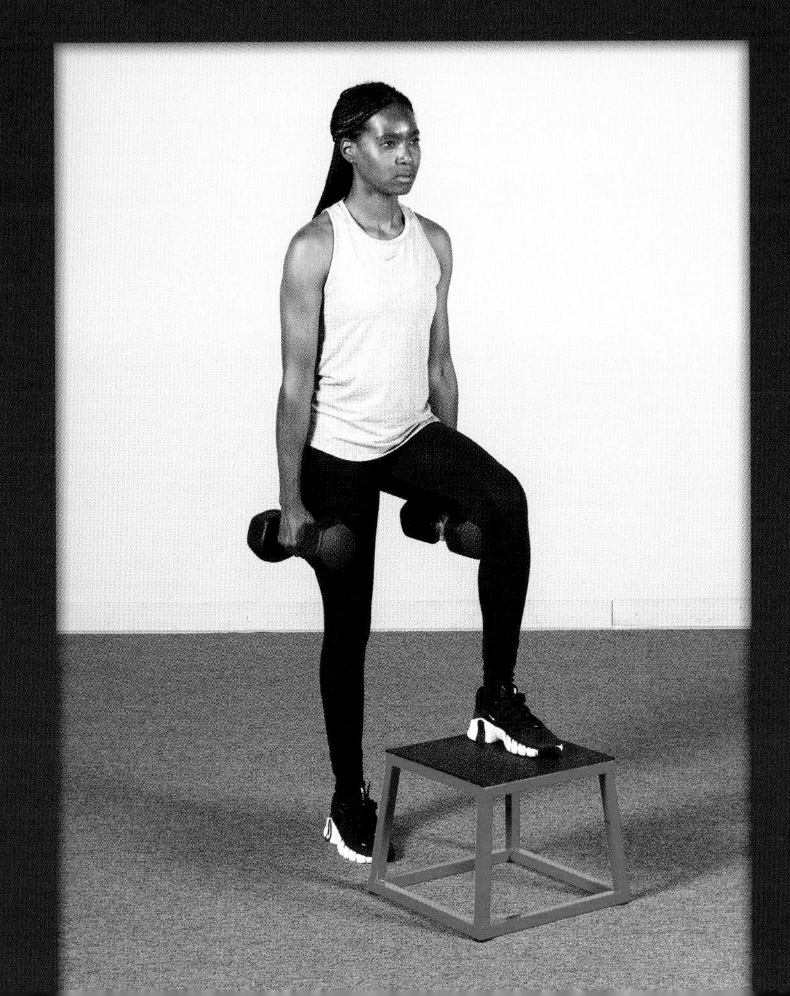

The lower-body exercises in this chapter are split up into two categories: knee dominant and hip dominant. Each category names the dominant joint to be moved, but most of the exercises recruit many different muscles in the lower body. A variety of squats and lunges focus on the quadriceps, hamstrings, and gluteus maximus as the prime muscles worked. Additionally, there are variations of squats and lunges in different planes of motion with different grips and handling of the weight. Be aware that when they are programmed into your workouts, how you hold the weight and where it is in relation to your body will matter. The different grips are described in the sidebar.

In the hip-dominant movements, you'll likely be hinging in a variation of a bridge on your back or standing in some sort of deadlift. "Hip dominant" also means that the hip takes precedence in the exercises. These movements focus more on the posterior muscle chain, with the hamstrings and glutei maximi being the prime muscles worked in the bridges and deadlifts, but you'll also work many other muscles. There are also some side-lying exercises using body weight that incorporate different movements with your legs, strengthening your hip adductors and abductors. These are essential in helping you move better with bigger lifts, like squats and deadlifts.

## VARIATION OF GRIPS FOR KNEE-DOMINANT AND HIP-DOMINANT EXERCISES

Goblet with dumbbell or kettlebell.

- Focus on keeping the dumbbell or kettlebell hugged in tight to your chest, with your elbows glued to your sides (*a*).

High goblet grip with dumbbell or kettlebell.

- Hold your elbows in line with your shoulders and keep your posture strong (*b*).
- The higher the dumbbell or kettlebell is, the more challenging it will be for your arms and core. You can hold the weight a little lower to make it less difficult.

Rack position with dumbbells.

- Keep each dumbbell in line with your shoulders and your elbows hugged in close to your rib cage (*c*).

Rack position with kettlebells.

- This is an advanced position.
- As the weight gets heavier, the back of your wrist will take some adjustment (*d*). It may be tender at first, but it may become less sore over time as you lift more frequently.
- Be mindful of wearable devices, watches, or jewelry, as the kettlebells can damage them.

Traditional front rack with barbell.

- Make sure the pins are in line with your armpits so that you are not tiptoeing back to the bar to rerack (*e*).
- Keep your elbows high.

Arms-crossed position with barbell

- Make sure the pins are in line with your armpits so that you are not tiptoeing back to the bar to rerack (*f*).
- Keep your elbows high.
- The arms-crossed position could be a good substitute if you have wrist issues or your flexibility is limited.

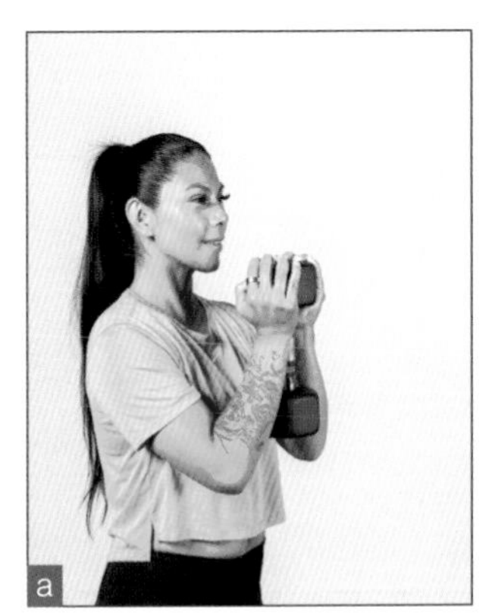
a

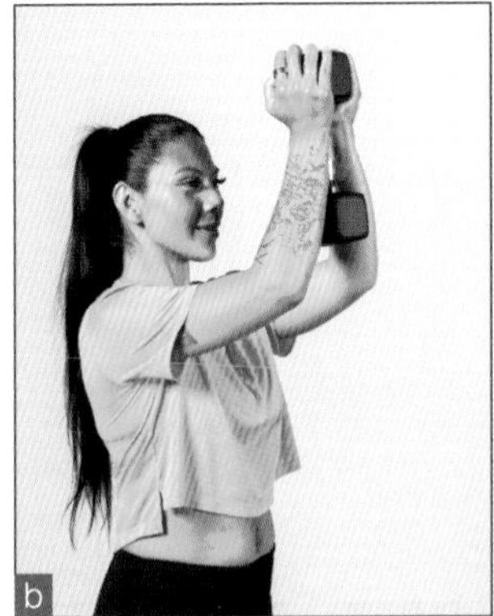
b

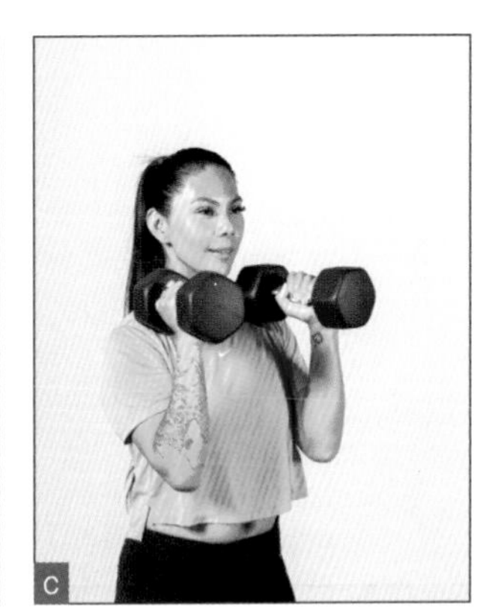
c

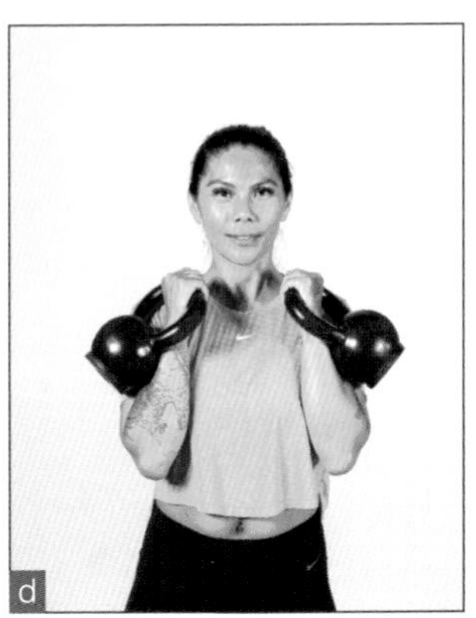
d

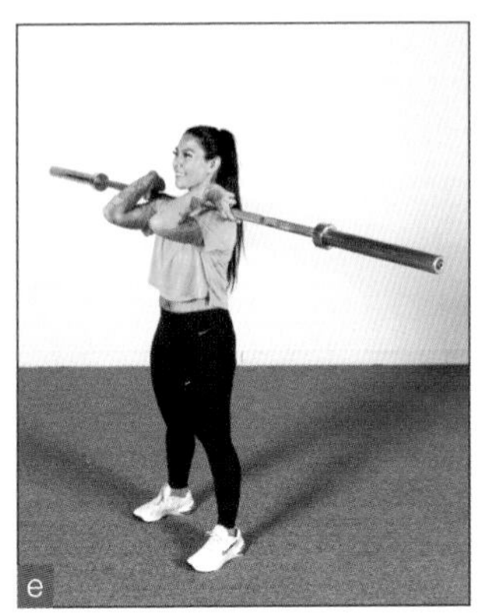
e

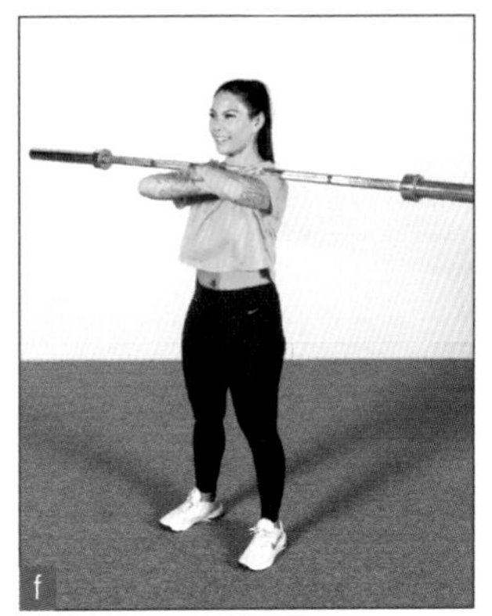
f

# GOBLET SQUAT

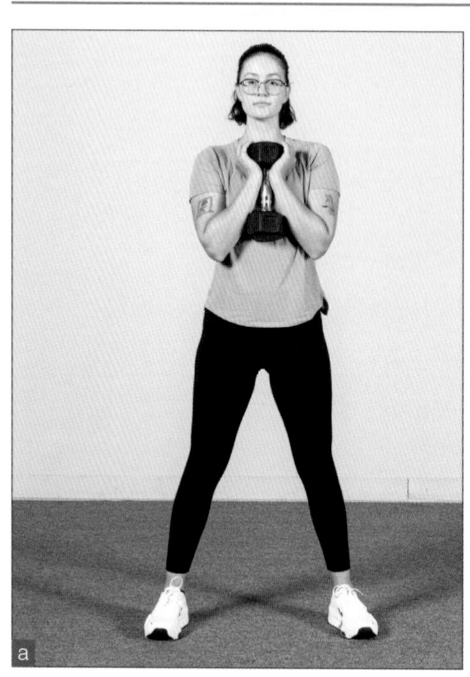
a

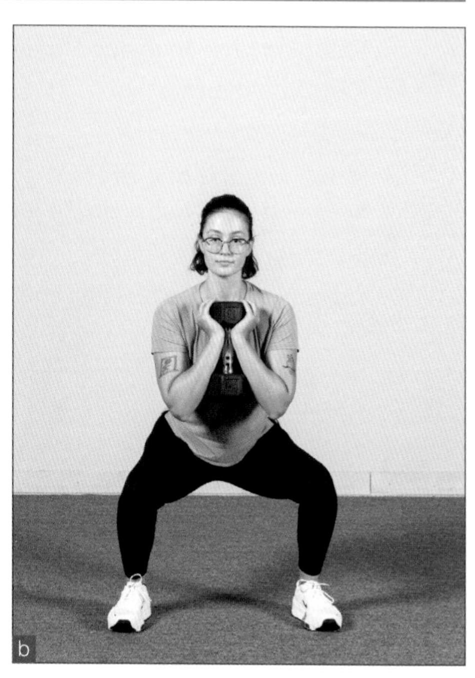
b

1. Stand with your feet about hip-width apart or just a little wider, holding one dumbbell with both hands and your elbows hugged in toward your rib cage (*a*).
2. Bend your knees, lowering your hips down to the ground, tracking your knees over your feet, keeping your posture tall (*b*).
3. Driving through your heels, straighten your legs to return to your starting position.

## Things to Keep in Mind

- Make sure that your feet are planted throughout the whole movement, so that your big toe, pinky toe, and heel are all pressing into the ground as you lower and stand.

## Variation

- The goblet squat can be done with high goblet grip or rack position with kettlebells or dumbbells.

# BACK SQUAT

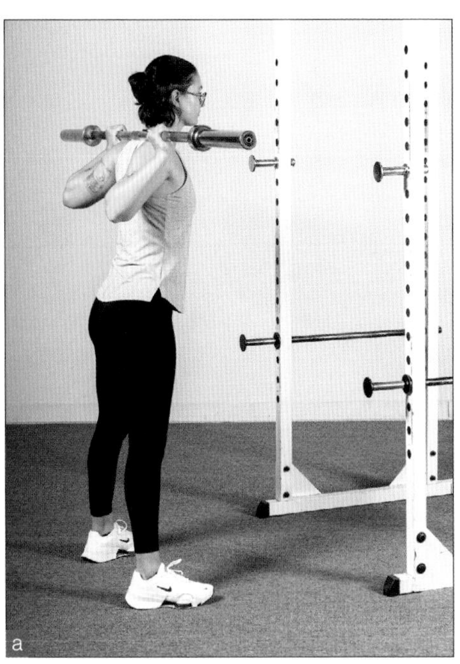
a

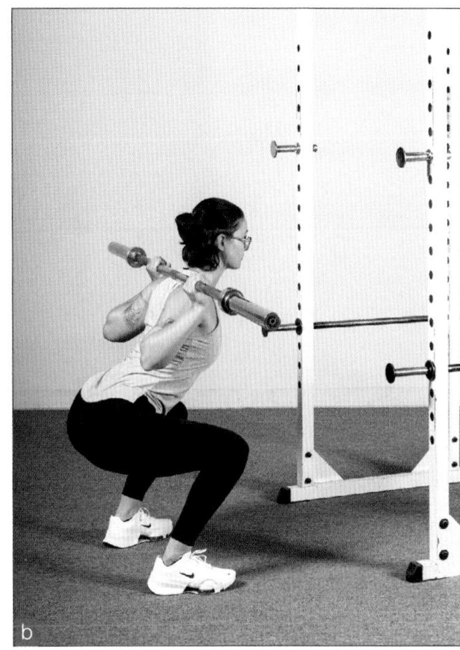
b

*Note:* A spotter may be needed.

1. Align yourself in front of a squat rack with the pins in line with your armpits.
2. With your knees bent slightly, walk yourself under the bar so that you feel pressure from the bar high on your shoulders.
3. Grip the bar with your palms facing away from you and elbows bent and lift the bar off the pins.
4. Once your grip feels steady, take a few steps away from the squat rack.
5. Ground your feet so they are about hip-width apart or just a little wider (*a*).
6. Bend your knees, lowering your hips to the ground, your knees over your feet, with your core engaged (*b*).
7. Driving through your heels, straighten your legs back to your starting position.
8. Complete the desired number of reps, then walk yourself back to the bar to safely rerack the weight.

## Things to Keep in Mind

- Make sure that your feet are planted throughout the whole movement, so that your big toe, pinky toe, and heel are all pressing into the ground as you lower and stand.
- Keep your neck in a neutral position throughout the movement; avoid looking up to the ceiling.

# TRADITIONAL FRONT RACK SQUAT

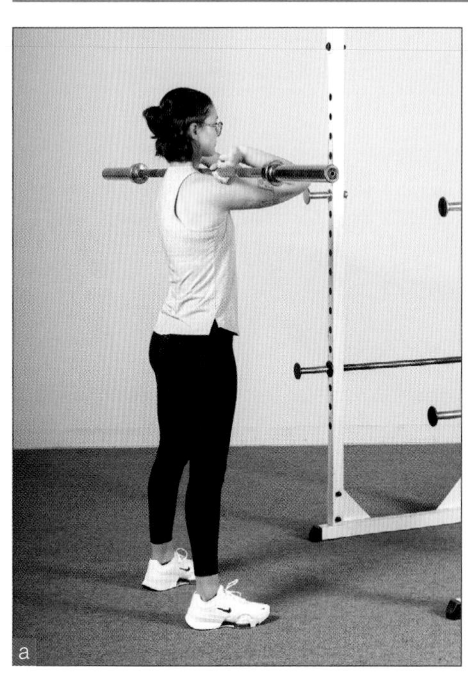
a

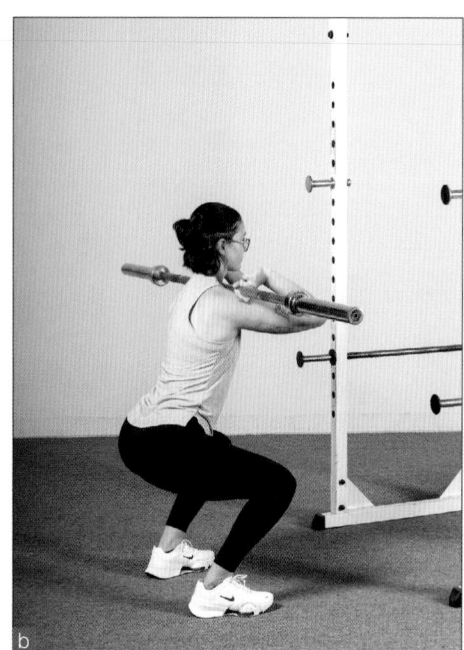
b

*Note*: A spotter may be needed.

1. Align yourself in front of a squat rack with the pins in line with your armpits.
2. Making sure that your knees are bent slightly, walk yourself to the bar so that you feel pressure from the bar high on your shoulders.
3. Bend your elbows and lift them high in line with your shoulders, hooking the first two fingers of each hand under the bar.
4. Once your grip feels steady, take a few steps away from the squat rack.
5. Ground your feet so they are about hip-width apart or just a little wider (*a*).
6. Bend your knees, lowering your hips to the ground, tracking your knees over your feet, with your core engaged (*b*).
7. Driving through your heels, straighten your legs to return to your starting position.
8. Complete the desired number of reps, then walk yourself back to the bar to safely rerack the weight.

## Things to Keep in Mind

- Make sure that your feet are planted throughout the whole movement, so that your big toe, pinky toe, and heel are all pressing into the ground as you lower and stand.
- Keep your neck in a neutral position throughout the movement; avoid looking up to the ceiling.

## POSTURE DIFFERENCE BETWEEN BACK SQUAT AND FRONT SQUAT OR GOBLET SQUAT

I favor front-loading squats over back-loading squats because front-loaded squatting movements tend to help you move with better postural integrity. This allows you to move more strongly through your squat with good form. Typically, you are able to load more when you are doing a back squat, so I always encourage learning a front squat first to ensure you have good form before moving onto the back squat.

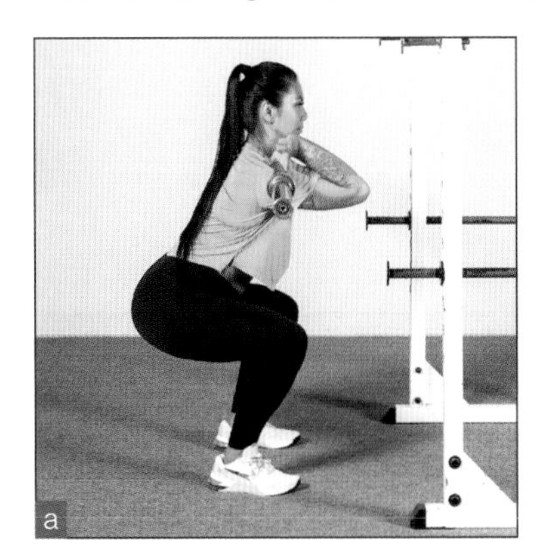

Front squat (side view): Holding the weight in front of you with your elbows high activates the front of your body and your core, keeping your posture more upright when you are at the bottom of the squat (*a*).

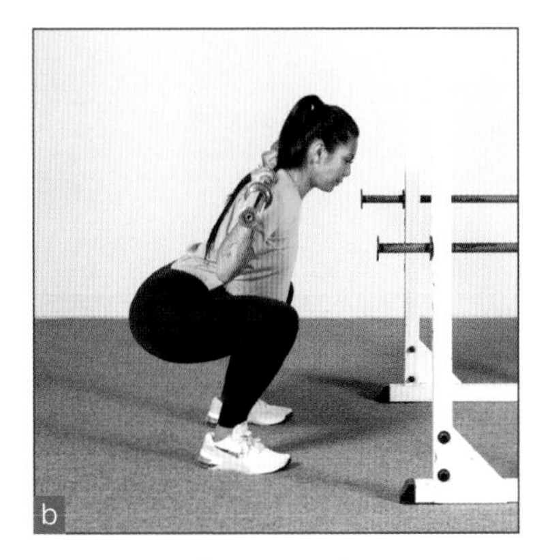

Back squat (side view): With the weight behind you, your chest will be a little more open, with a little rib flare. You may have a slight forward lean at the bottom of the squat (*b*).

# GOBLET STAGGERED SQUAT

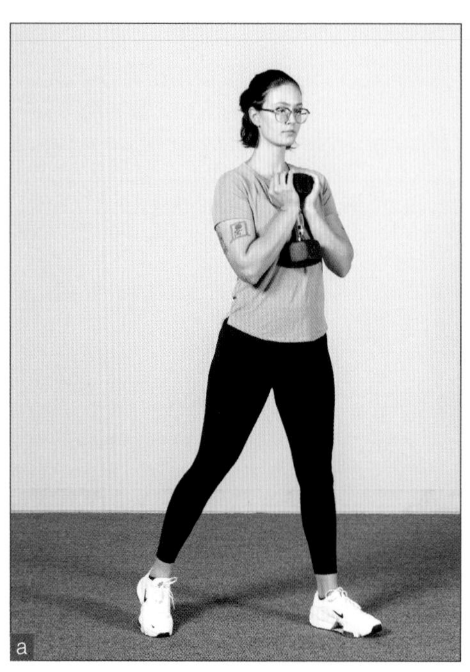
a

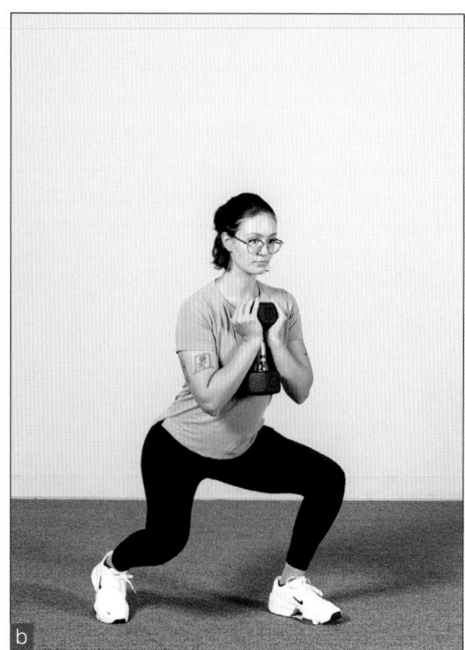
b

1. Stand with your feet about hip-width apart or just a little wider, holding one dumbbell in both hands in front of your chest, with your elbows hugged in toward your rib cage.
2. Slide one foot back a few inches so that your toe is in line with the back of your front foot with your heel lifted (*a*).
3. Bend your knees, lowering your hips down to the ground with your hips squared forward and weight evenly distributed through both sides (*b*).
4. Keep your posture tall as you lower down.
5. Drive through your front foot and the ball of your back foot to straighten your legs and return to your starting position.
6. Complete the desired number of reps and repeat on the other side.

## Things to Keep in Mind

- Pretend you have headlights on your hips that must shine straight ahead.

## Variation

- The goblet staggered squat can be done with high goblet grip or rack position with kettlebells or dumbbells.

# GOBLET SUMO SQUAT

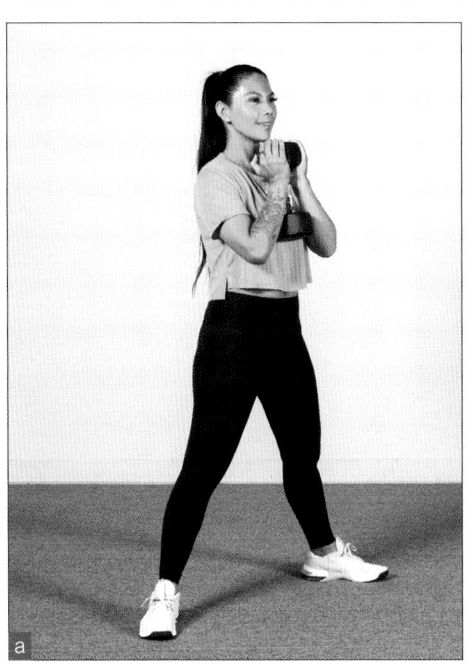


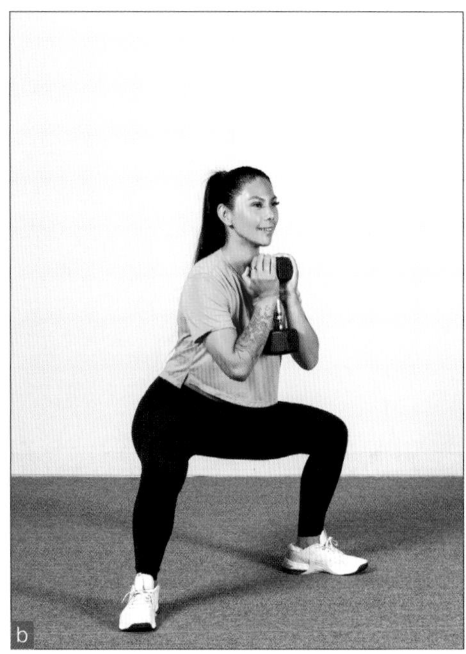


1. Stand with your feet wider than your hips and your toes turned out, holding one dumbbell in both hands in front of your chest, with your elbows hugged in toward your rib cage (*a*).
2. Bend your knees, lowering your hips toward the ground, keeping your posture tall (*b*).
3. Drive through your feet to straighten your legs back and return to your starting position.
4. Complete the desired number of repetitions.

## Things to Keep in Mind

- Do your best to keep your knees in line with your feet, making sure that each foot is solidly planted.

## Variation

- The goblet sumo squat can be done with high goblet grip or rack position with kettlebells or dumbbells.

# WALL SIT

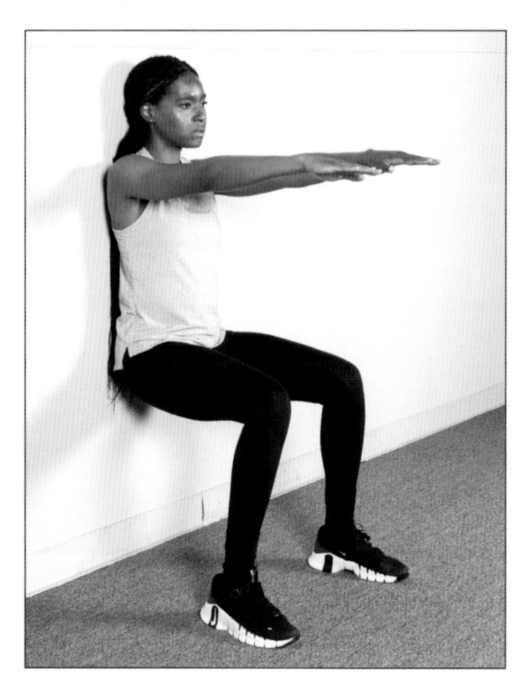

1. With your back against a sturdy wall and your feet about hip-width apart, walk your feet out in front of you as you slide your back down the wall, bending your knees so that your thighs are parallel to the ground or your hips are a little lower than your knees.
2. You can rest your hands gently on your thighs or hold them straight out in front of you for an added challenge.
3. Hold for the desired amount of time.

## Things to Keep in Mind

- Keep your shoulders against the wall the whole time.
- Do not allow your heels or toes to come off the ground.

# DUMBBELL REVERSE LUNGE

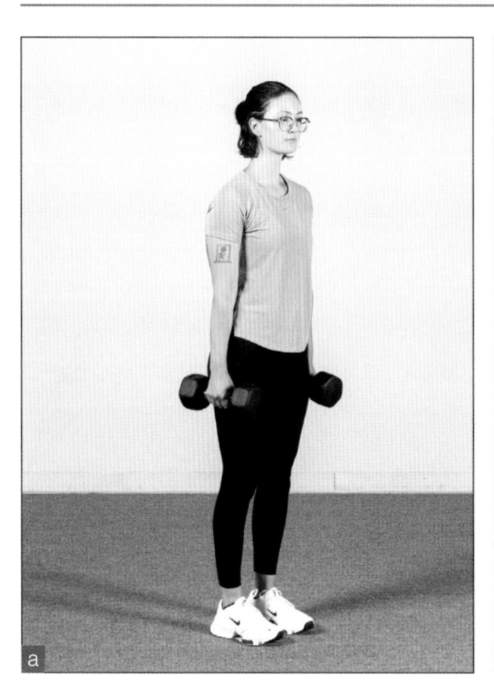

a

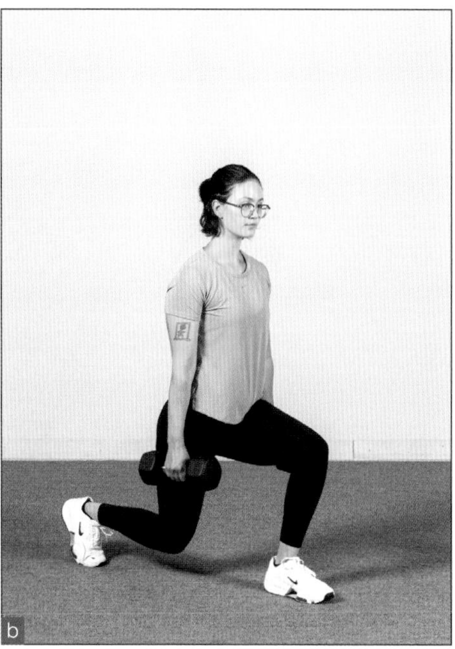

b

1. Stand with your feet hip-width apart, holding a dumbbell in each hand (*a*).
2. Step one foot back far enough back to where you can bend your knees.
3. Keep your hips squared forward as you bend your knees, lowering your back knee to the ground (*b*).
4. Drive through your front foot to return to your starting position.
5. Complete the desired number of reps and then repeat on the other side, or alternate sides.

## Things to Keep in Mind

- Keep your posture upright, allowing a full extension in your back hip.
- Make sure you are not stepping back as though you were on a tightrope; keep some space laterally between the feet.

## Variations

- The dumbbell reverse lunge can be done with high goblet grip or rack position with kettlebells or dumbbells. It can also be done as a body-weight exercise.
- This exercise can also be done with arms overhead for an advanced option for stability and mobility.

# DUMBBELL FORWARD LUNGE

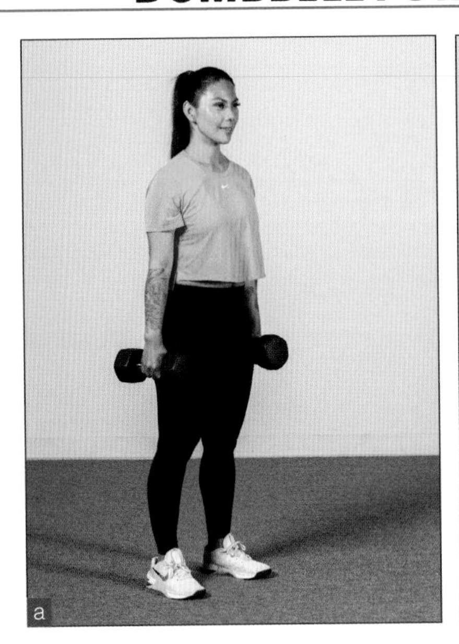

a

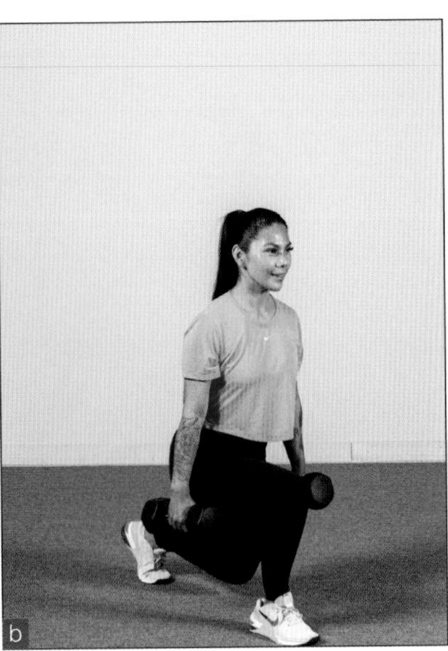

b

1. Stand with your feet hip-width apart, holding a dumbbell in each hand (*a*).
2. Step one foot forward enough to where you can bend your knees.
3. Keep your hips squared forward as you bend your knees, lowering your back knee to the ground (*b*).
4. Drive through your front foot to return to your starting position.
5. Complete the desired number of reps and then repeat on the other side, or alternate sides.

## Things to Keep in Mind

- The forward lunge is more challenging than the reverse lunge; use a smaller range of motion if needed and don't lowering your knee as much.
- Keep your posture upright, allowing a full extension in your back hip.
- Make sure you are not stepping forward as though you were on a tightrope.

## Variations

- The dumbbell forward lunge can be done with high goblet grip or rack position with kettlebells or dumbbells.
- This exercise can also be done with arms overhead for an advanced option for stability and mobility.

## SPLIT SQUAT VERSUS STATIONARY LUNGE

They're the same movement, so why the two different names?

"Squat" connotes one foot or two feet planted while the knee bends, with no forward or backward motion. Lunges are typically understood to entail motion. Technically, therefore, the term "stationary lunge" is illogical, and this is why one move has two different names!

# DUMBBELL STATIONARY LUNGE OR SPLIT SQUAT

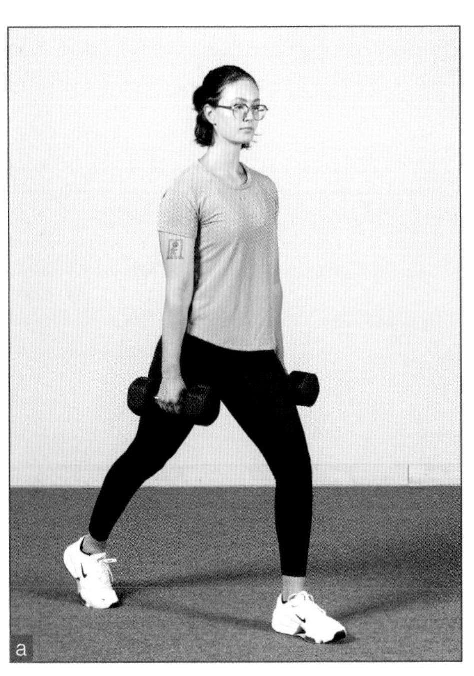

a

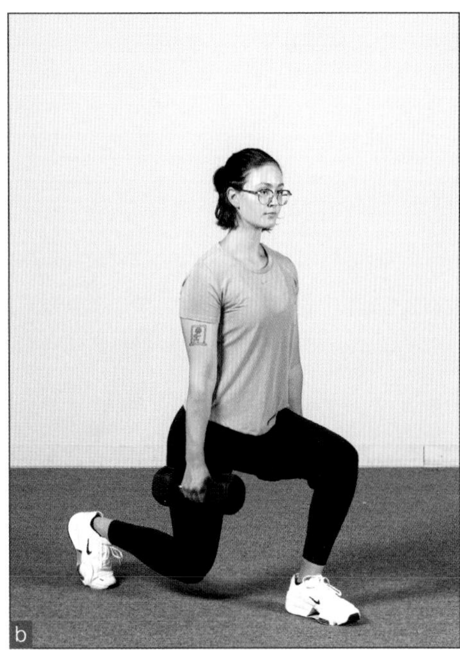

b

1. Stand with one foot forward and the other foot back, as if you were in a lunge, with your back heel lifted and a dumbbell in each hand (*a*).
2. Keep your feet planted and hips squared forward as you bend your knees, lowering your back knee toward the ground (*b*).
3. Continue to keep both feet planted and straighten your knees to bring you back to your starting position.
4. Complete the desired number of reps, and then repeat on the other side.

## Things to Keep in Mind

- Attempt only the range of motion that feels good for you.
- Make sure your feet are not in line as though you were on a tightrope, but that they are hip-width apart.
- Pretend you have headlights on your hips that must shine straight ahead. Do not allow your hips to turn out.

## Variation

- The dumbbell stationary lunge or split squat can be done with goblet grip or rack position with kettlebells or dumbbells.

# DUMBBELL BULGARIAN SPLIT SQUAT OR REAR FOOT ELEVATED SPLIT SQUAT

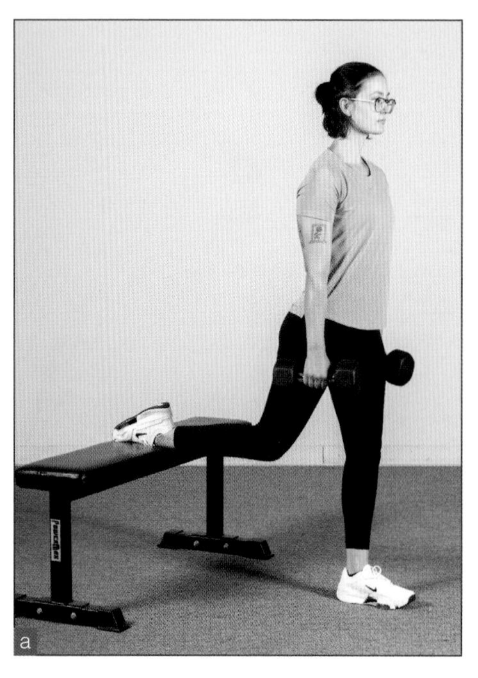

a

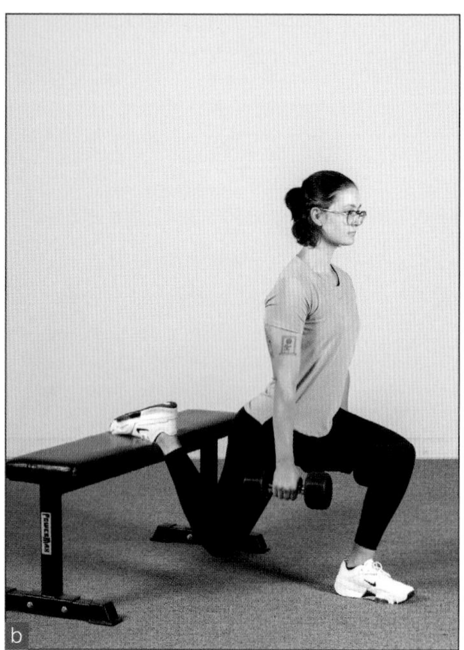

b

1. Stand 12 to 18 inches (30.48-45.72 cm) away from a bench or single-leg roller stand, facing away from it, holding a dumbbell in each hand.
2. Lower into a half-kneeling position, with one knee on the ground.
3. Place your back foot on the bench or single-leg roller stand, with the top of your foot flat on the surface.
4. Square your hips forward and press down into your front foot to stand. This is your starting position (*a*).
5. Bend both knees to slowly lower your back knee toward the ground, keeping your knee off the ground to the lowest point at which you feel comfortable (*b*).
6. Complete the desired number of reps, and then repeat on the other side.

## Things to Keep in Mind

- Make sure that your back leg isn't too high; adjust as necessary and attempt only the range of motion that feels good for you.
- Make sure your feet are not in line as though you were on a tightrope, but that they are hip distance apart.
- Pretend you have headlights on your hips that must shine straight ahead. Do not allow your hips to turn out.

## Variation

- The dumbbell Bulgarian split squat or rear foot elevated split squat can be done with high goblet grip or rack position with kettlebells or dumbbells.

# DUMBBELL STEP-UP

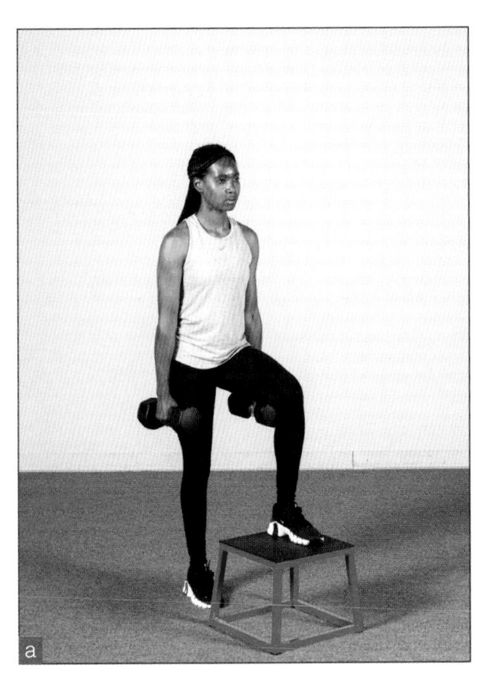
a

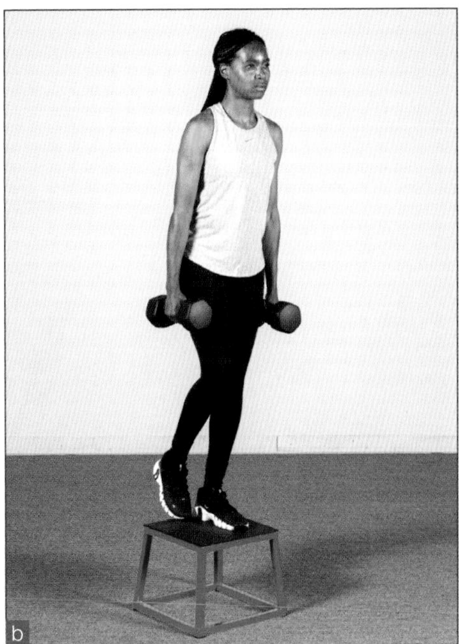
b

1. Stand facing a box that is 12 to 18 inches (30.48-45.72 cm) high, holding a dumbbell in each hand.
2. Step forward, placing one foot on the box (*a*).
3. Keep your hips forward and your core engaged as you push through the foot on the box to bring yourself upright on top of the box (*b*).
4. Tap your back foot to the box and lower that same foot to the starting position.
5. Complete the desired number of reps and then repeat on the other side, or alternate sides.

## Things to Keep in Mind

- Make sure that your back isn't rounding as you step up on the box; use a shorter box or a lighter weight if necessary.
- Use the leg on top of the box to push yourself up, rather than pushing off the floor with the back foot.

## Variation

- The dumbbell step-up can be done with goblet grip or rack position with kettlebells or dumbbells.

# DUMBBELL LATERAL LUNGE

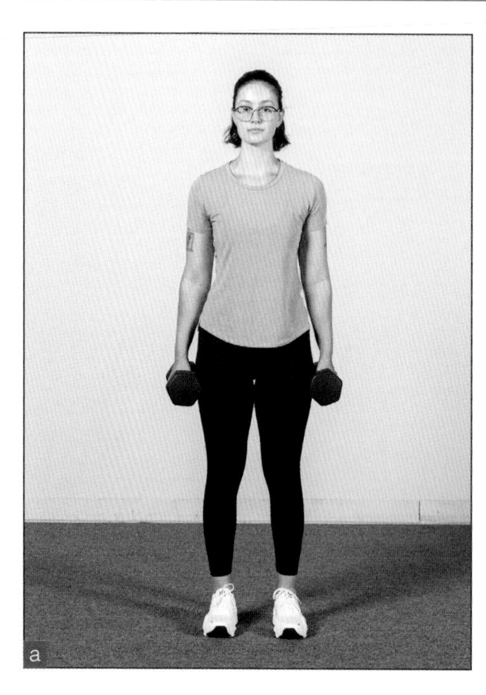
a

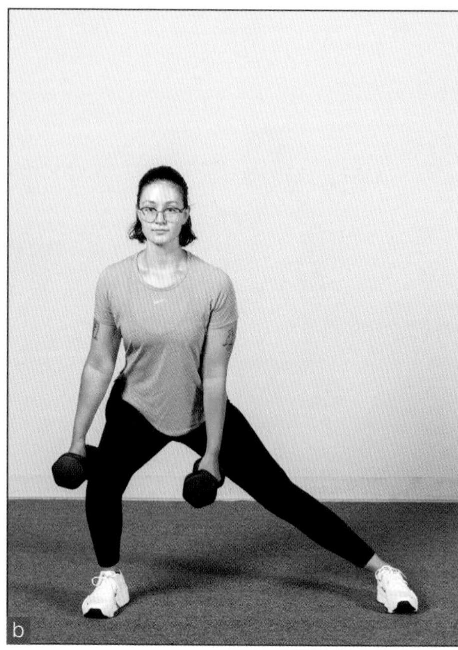
b

1. Stand with both feet about hip-width apart, feet pointing forward, holding a dumbbell in each hand (*a*).
2. Step one foot to the side, keeping your posture tall and toes facing forward, framing your knee with a dumbbell on each side.
3. Bend the knee of the foot that has stepped out to the side while sinking into that hip and simultaneously straightening the opposite leg (*b*).
4. Push through the foot that has stepped out to bring you back to your starting position.
5. Complete the desired number of reps and then repeat on the other side, or alternate sides.

## Things to Keep in Mind

- Try not to step out too far and overstretch.
- Pretend there are headlights on your hips that must shine straight ahead as you move side to side.

## Variations

- The dumbbell lateral lunge can be done with goblet grip or rack position with kettlebells or dumbbells.
- This can also be done as a stationary exercise: start with your feet wide; stay planted and shift your weight side to side for the lateral lunge position.

# DUMBBELL CURTSY LUNGE

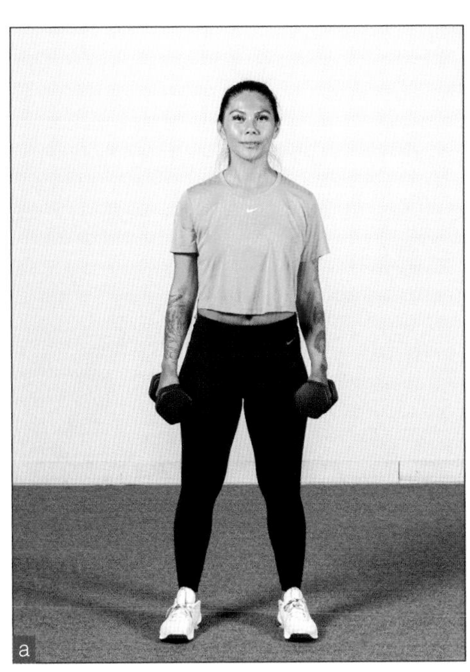

a

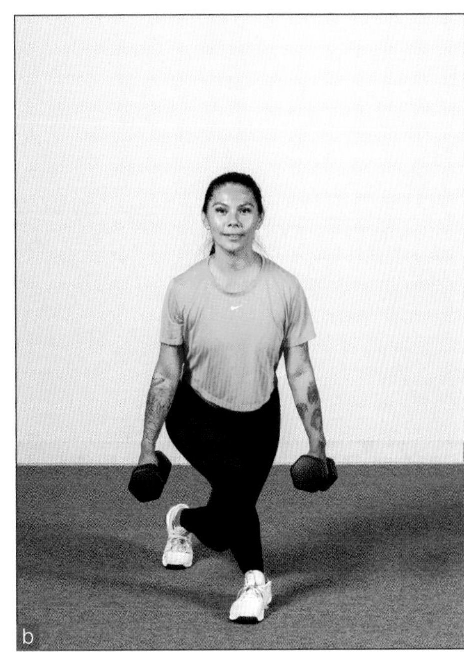

b

1. Stand with your feet pointing forward, about hip-width apart, holding a dumbbell in each hand (*a*).
2. Step one foot back and behind the other leg; go just far enough to keep your hips squared forward, holding the dumbbells at your sides.
3. Bend both of your knees and lower yourself as close to the floor as is comfortable given your range of motion (*b*).
4. Drive through the front foot to return to your starting position.
5. Complete the desired number of reps and then repeat on the other side, or alternate sides.

## Things to Keep in Mind

- Try not to step back too far;, move only through the range of motion that is comfortable.
- Pretend there are headlights on your hips that must shine straight ahead as you move side to side.

## Variation

- The dumbbell curtsy lunge can be done with high goblet grip or rack position with kettlebells or dumbbells.

# DUMBBELL BACK DIAGONAL LUNGE

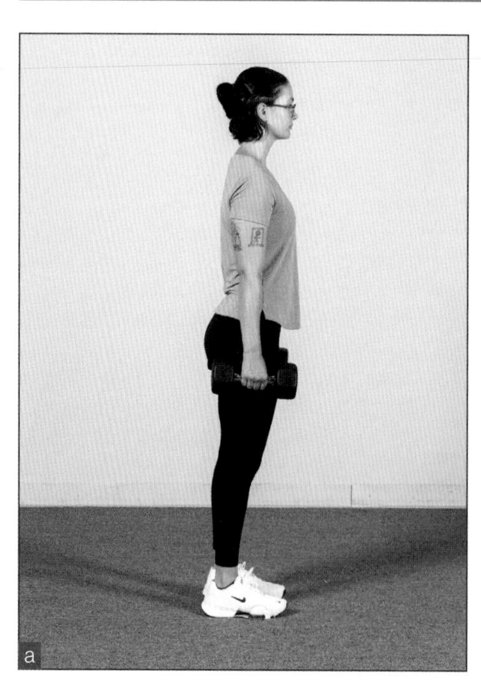
a

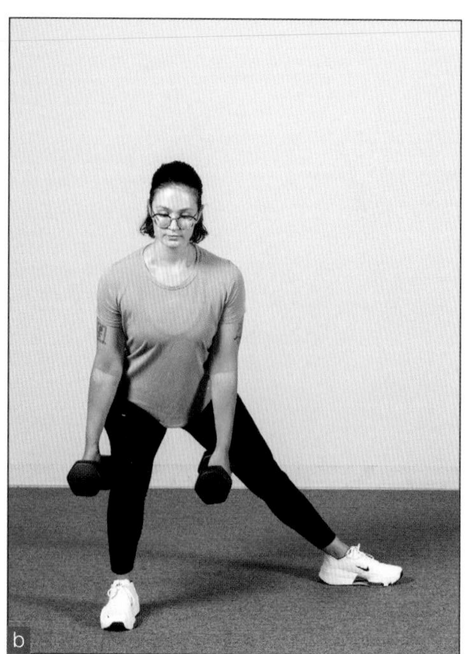
b

1. Stand with your feet about hip-width apart and pointing forward, with a dumbbell in each hand (*a*).
2. Keep one foot grounded as you turn your body and step the other foot diagonally behind you, bending that knee and keeping your other leg straight, framing your knee with a dumbbell on each side (*b*).
3. Keep your core engaged and posture up as you sink into the hip of the side that stepped diagonally back.
4. Drive through that same foot to return to your starting position.
5. Complete the desired number of reps and then repeat on the other side, or alternate sides.

## Things to Keep in Mind

- Think of this move like a lateral lunge that is moving to the back corner.
- Try not to step back too far and overstretch; you should move your foot to the back ever so slightly.

## Variation

- The dumbbell back diagonal lunge can be done with high goblet grip or rack position with kettlebells or dumbbells.

# BRIDGE

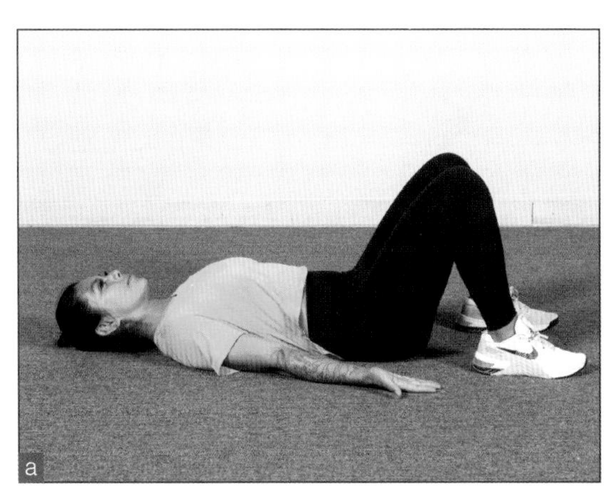
a

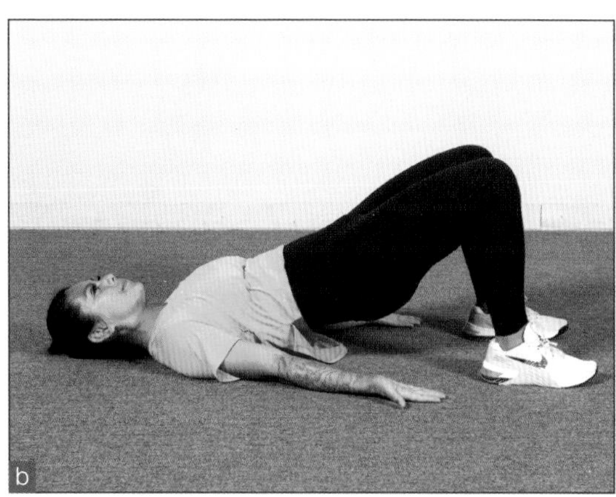
b

1. Lie on your back with your knees bent and your feet a few inches away from your butt, arms at your side with your palms facing up (*a*).
2. Push your heels into the ground as you lift your hips up toward the sky, pressing the backs of your hands into the floor (*b*).
3. Focus on keeping your tailbone tucked and rib cage in.
4. Hold for 1 to 2 seconds or the desired amount of time, then lower your hips back to the starting position.
5. Complete the desired number of reps.

## Things to Keep in Mind

- Higher is not better on this movement. Avoid extending your lower back.
- Focus on keeping your pelvis tucked and not letting your lower back arch as you press up.

## Variations

### Barbell or Dumbbell Bridge

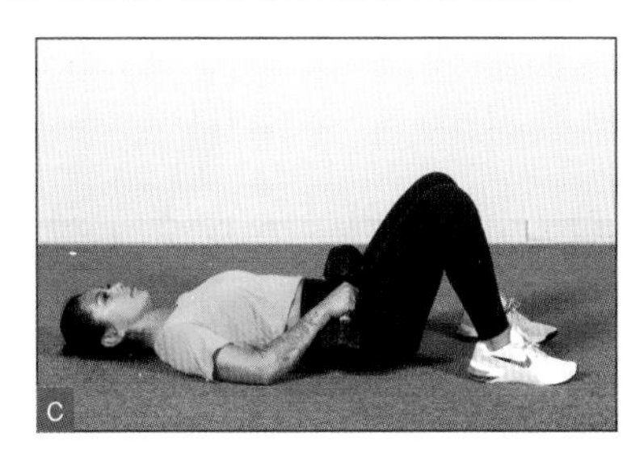
c

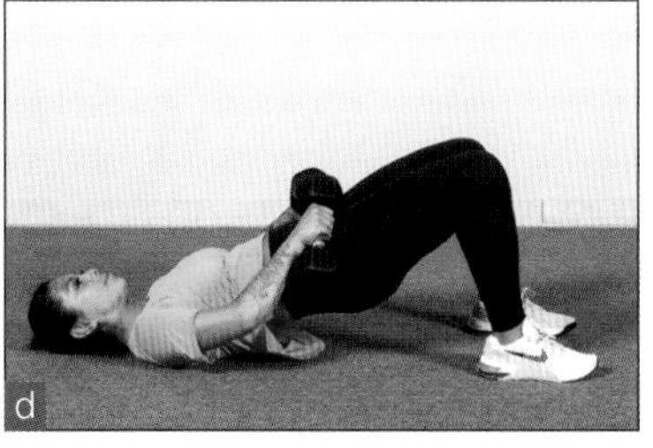
d

1. Lie on your back with your knees bent and your feet a few inches away from your butt, and one or two dumbbells (*c*) or a barbell sitting along the crease of your hip.
2. Repeat steps 2 through 5 of the bridge exercise (*d*).

Hip Dominant

## Single-Leg Bridge

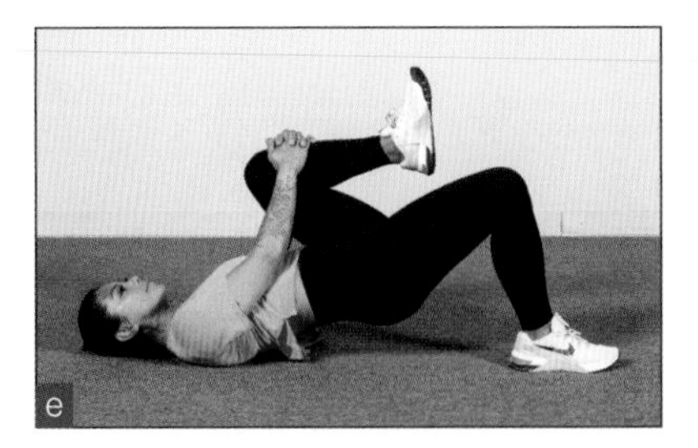
e

1. Lie on your back as you would for a bridge, then lift one leg off the ground, bring your knee toward your chest, and wrap your hands around your shin to hug your knee into your chest.
2. Push the heel that is on the floor into the ground to drive your hips up toward the ceiling, the pause for a second (or for the desired amount of time, if a hold; *e*).
3. Lower down slowly, and complete the desired amount of repetitions. Repeat on the other side.

## Long Bridge

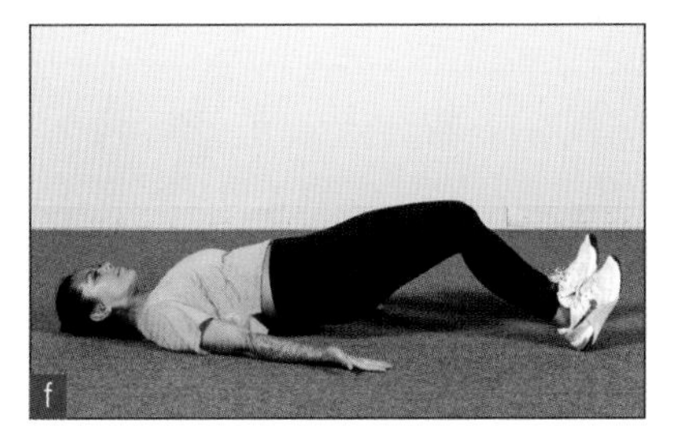
f

1. Lie on your back like you would for a bridge, but step your heels out slightly farther than they would be for a regular bridge (*f*).
2. Repeat steps 2 through 5 of bridge.

## Staggered Bridge

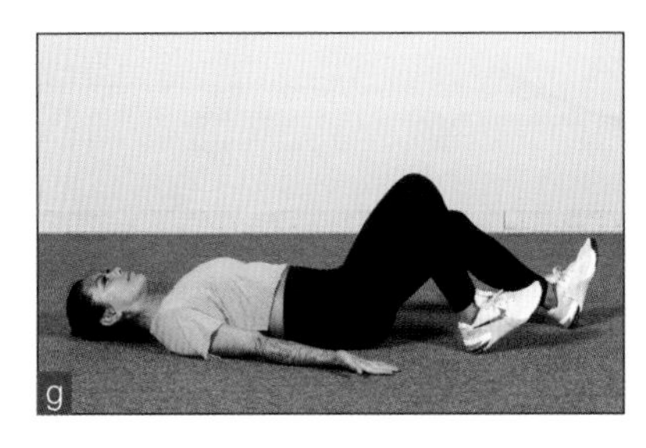
g

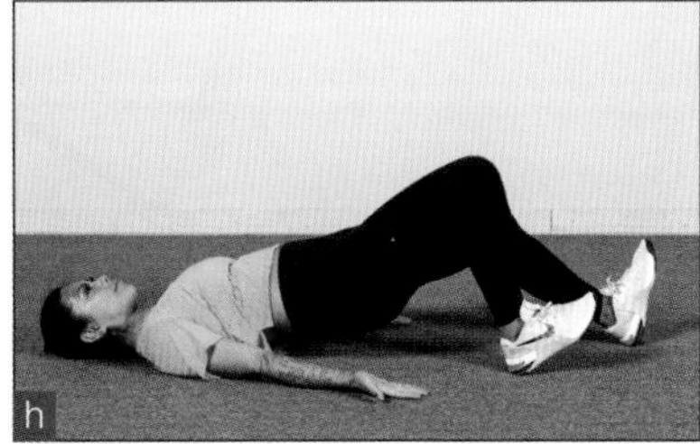
h

1. Lie on your back like you would for a bridge, but step one heel out a just a little bit (*g*).
2. Repeat steps 2 through 4 of bridge (*h*).

## BARBELL HIP THRUST

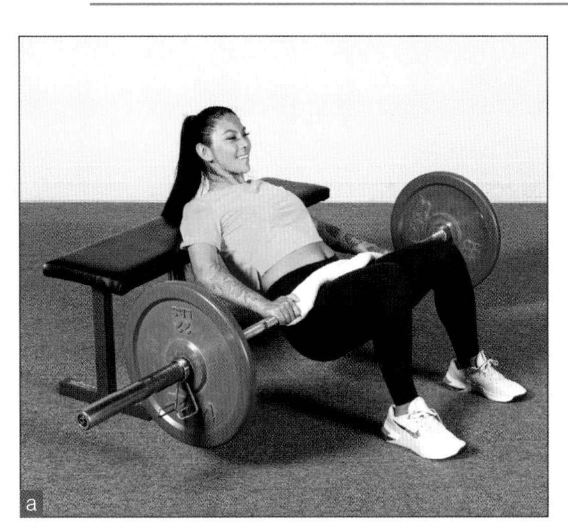
a

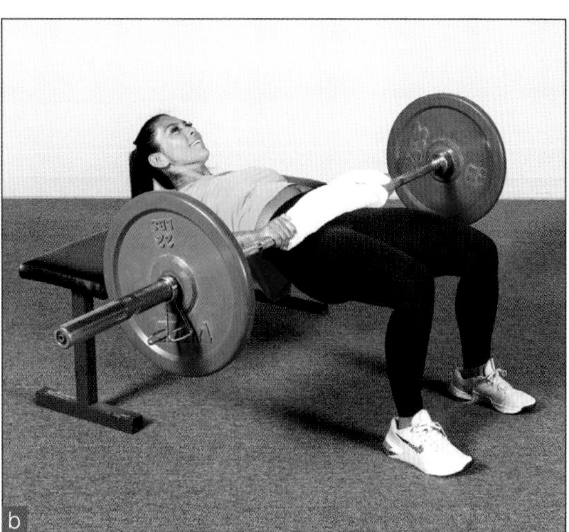
b

1. Sit with your back against a sturdy box or bench that is about the height of your knees, and place a barbell across your hips (you can pad the barbell to add comfort with a pad or rolled up towel; *a*).
2. Bend your knees so that your feet are a few inches away from your butt.
3. Press your back into the box or bench so that your shoulder blades are just above the edge of the box, while simultaneously pressing your heels into the floor and holding the barbell with both hands to guide it.
4. Push your hips up toward the sky, keeping your chin tucked as you let your back hinge onto the box or bench (*b*).
5. Hold for 1 to 2 seconds or for desired amount of time, making sure you keep your rib cage in and tailbone tucked.
6. Lower your hips back down to the ground slowly, and complete the desired number of reps.

### Things to Keep in Mind

- Higher is not better on this movement. Avoid extending your lower back.
- Focus on keeping your pelvis tucked and not letting your lower back arch as you press up.

### Variation

- The barbell hip thrust can be done with body weight as a hold or dumbbells.

## Staggered Barbell Hip Thrust

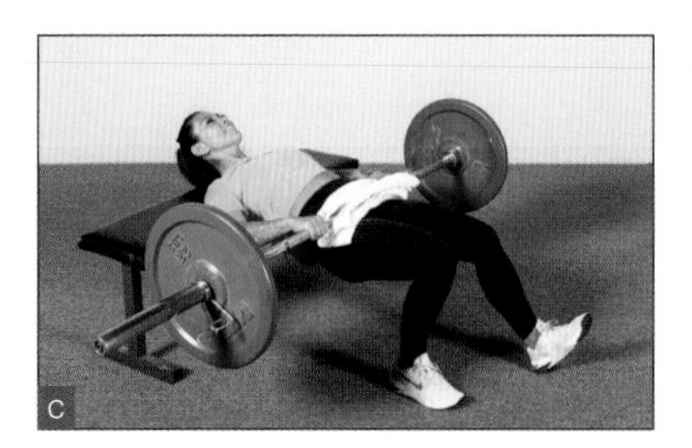
c

1. Sit with your back against a sturdy box or bench that is about the height of your knees, and place a barbell across your hips (you can pad the barbell to add comfort).
2. Bend your knees so that your feet are a few inches away from your butt, but stagger one foot 6 to 8 inches (15.24-20.32 cm) in front of the other; raise the toes of the front foot off the ground and let the heel dig into the ground (*c*).
3. Repeat steps 3 through 6 of the barbell hip thrust. Complete the desired number of reps. Repeat on the other side.

This variation can be done with body weight or dumbbells.

## ROMANIAN DEADLIFT VERSUS CONVENTIONAL OR AMERICAN DEADLIFT

Deadlift exercises work the back side of your body, or your posterior chain, with a focus on your glutes, hamstrings, core, and back. The biggest difference between the Romanian deadlift and the conventional or American deadlift is how they start and end. When you hear a lifter refer to "deadlifts," it's likely they are talking about the conventional or American deadlift. This movement is exactly what it sounds like: lifting "dead weight" from the ground. The weight is heavy. You hinge at your hips to start, then stand up and pick up the weight, and then lower it back down and reset between reps (*a*). In the Romanian deadlift, the weight starts in front of your quadriceps. You hinge at your hips when you lower the weight, then stand back up (*b*). You'll be gripping the weight for the entirety of the set, so the weight you choose should be lighter than a traditional deadlift.

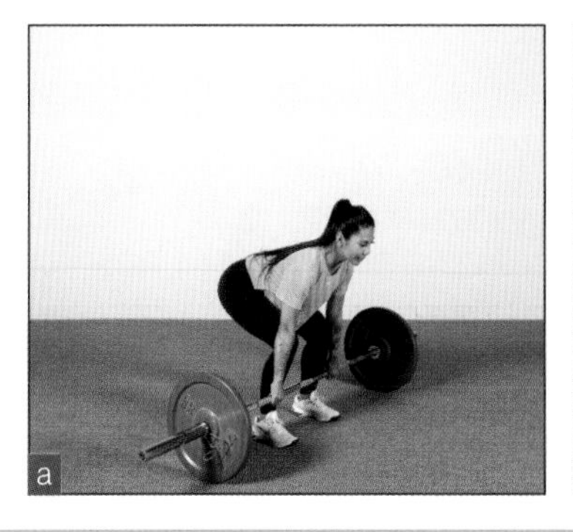
a

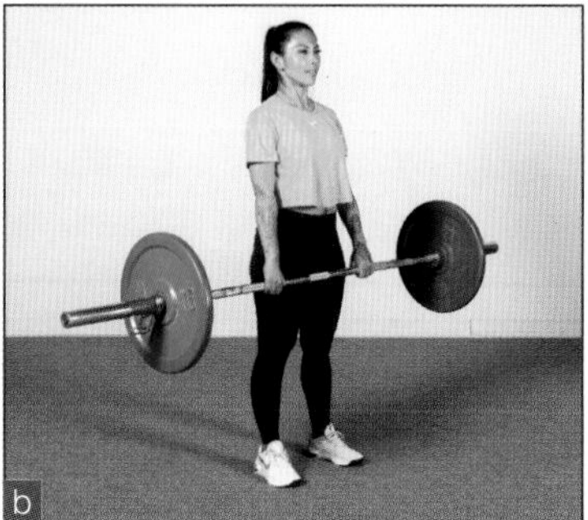
b

# ROMANIAN DEADLIFT

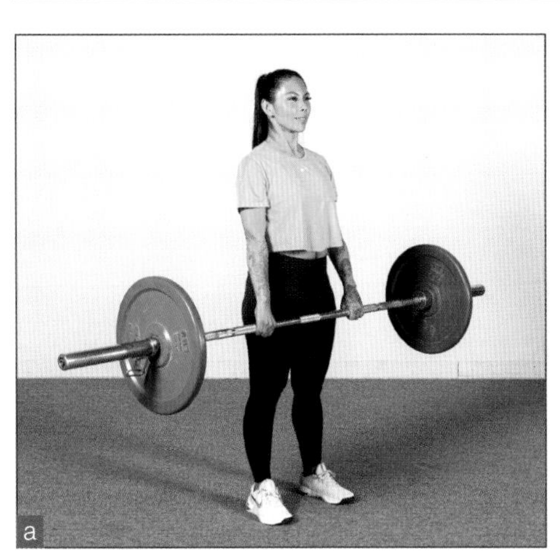


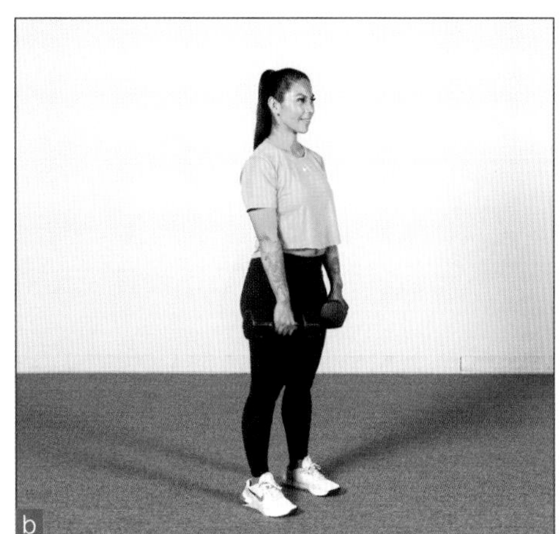


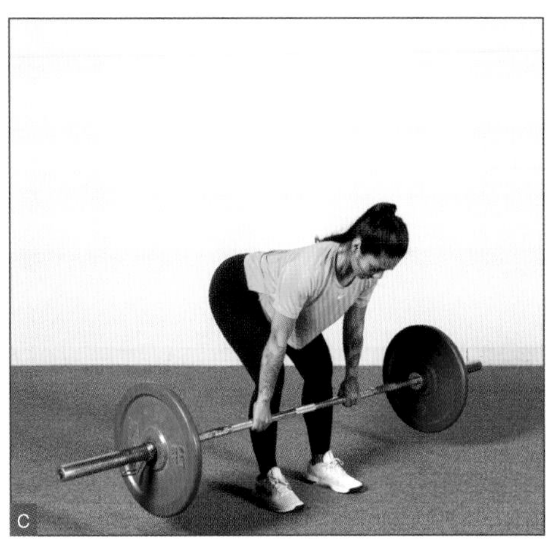


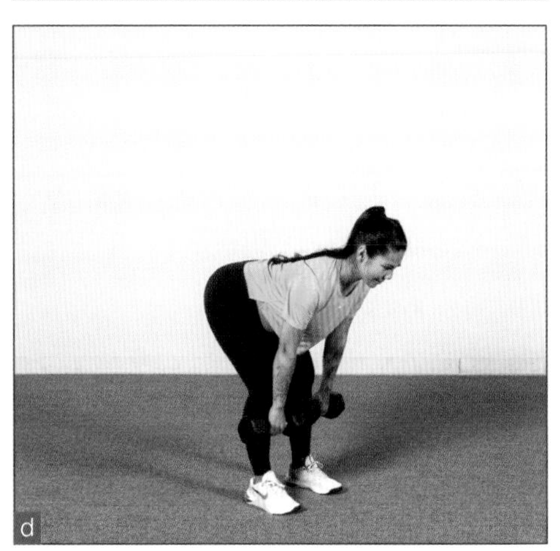


1. Stand with both feet under your hips and your knees slightly bent. With both arms straight, hold the barbell (*a*) or dumbbells (*b*) in front of your thighs.
2. Keep your spine long and chin tucked as you hinge at your hips, moving your hips back behind you.
3. Slide your barbell (*c*) or dumbbells (*d*) down your legs, going only as far as you can to the point at which you can keep your core engaged.
4. Hold at the end range of motion where your core is engaged for 1 to 2 seconds or for the desired amount of time.
5. Return to your starting position, and complete the desired number of reps.

## Things to Keep in Mind

- Do not lock your knees. Make sure they are slightly bent for the whole exercise.
- Lower is not better with this movement. If your back starts to round, you lose engagement with your core.
- Attempt only the range of motion that feels good to you.
- Do not lean back or extend your lower back when you stand up.

## Variation

## Staggered Romanian Deadlift

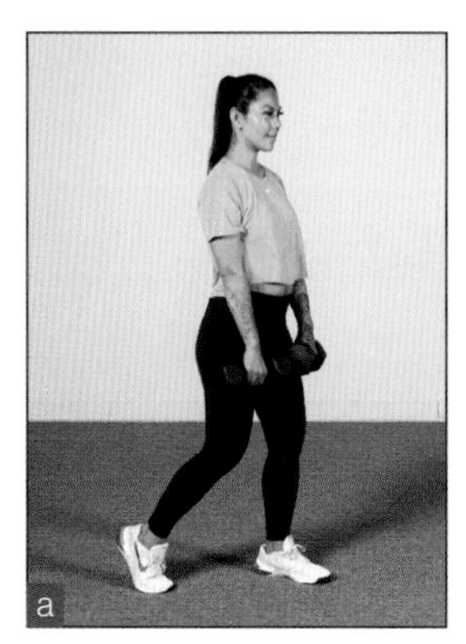
a

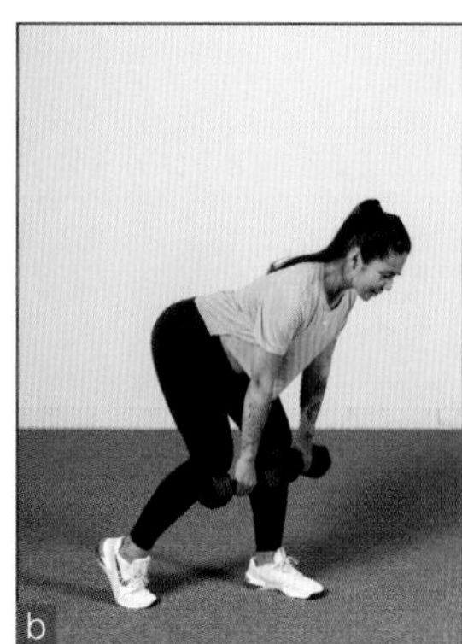
b

1. Stand with both feet under your hips and your knees slightly bent.
2. Slide one foot back so that heel is lifted and those toes are in line with your other heel.
3. Keep a soft bend in both knees, and hold your weight in front of your thighs, keeping your hips squared forward (*e*).
4. Repeat steps 3 through 5 of Romanian deadlift (*f*).

## Things to Keep in Mind

- Let your back foot be a kickstand, allowing your front foot to bear most of your weight.
- Do not lock your knees. Make sure they are slightly bent for the whole exercise.
- Lower is not better with this movement. If your back starts to round, you lose engagement with your core.
- Attempt only the range of motion that feels good to you.
- Do not lean back or extend your lower back when you stand up.

## SINGLE-LEG ROMANIAN DEADLIFT

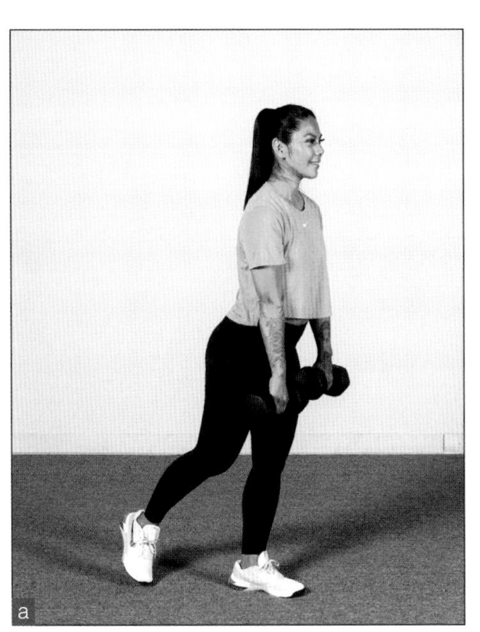

a

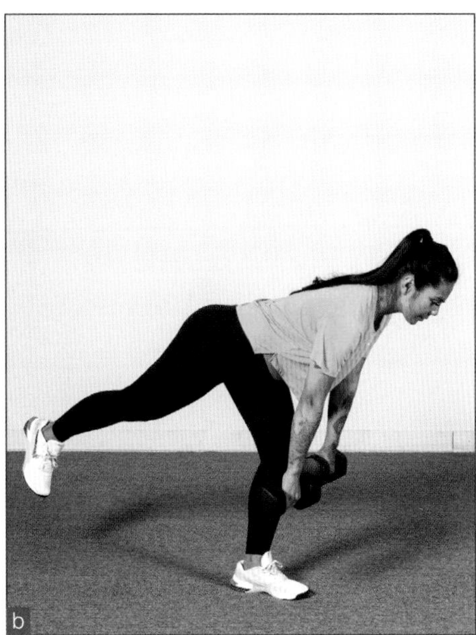

b

1. Stand on one foot with your knee slightly bent and your other leg off the floor and slightly behind you.
2. Hold your dumbbells or barbell in front of your thighs with your hips squared forward (*a*).
3. Keep your spine long and chin tucked as you hinge at your hips, moving your hips back and allowing your trailing leg to come up in line with your spine as you hinge and slide your weights down your legs (*b*).
4. Go only as far as you can while keeping your core engaged. Hold the end range of motion for 1 to 2 seconds or the desired amount of time.
5. Slowly stand back up, lowering your trailing leg to return to the start position.
6. Reset your feet and posture and complete the desired number of reps.
7. Repeat on the other leg.

### Things to Keep in Mind

- Do not lock your knees. Make sure they are slightly bent for the whole exercise.
- Lower is not better with this movement. If your back starts to round, you lose engagement with your core.
- Attempt only the range of motion that feels good to you.
- Do not lean back or extend your lower back when you stand up.

# GOOD MORNING

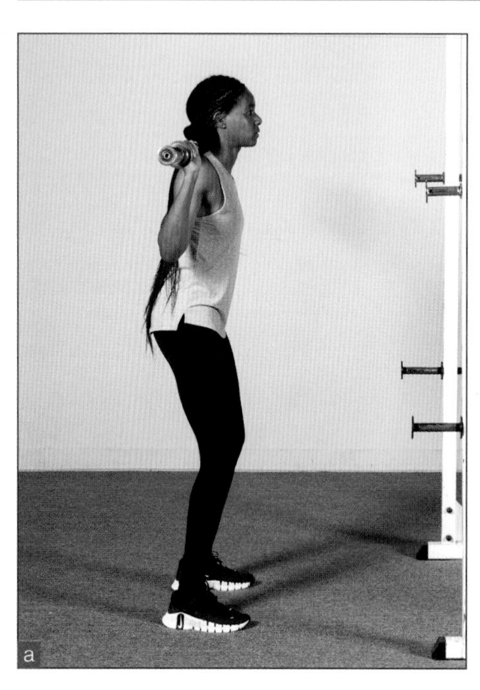
a

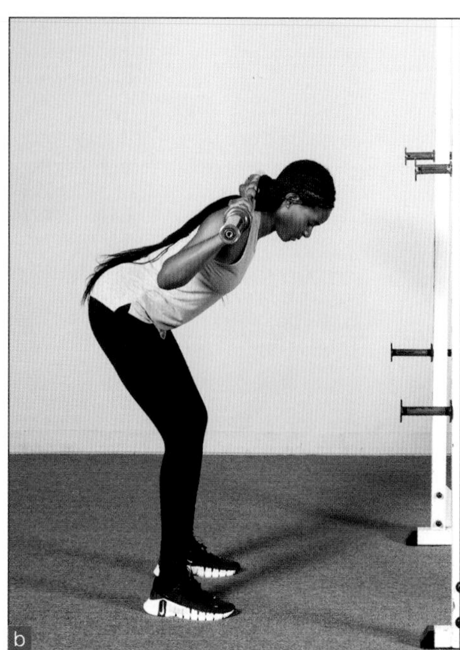
b

1. Stand in front of a squat rack with the pins and bar in line a few inches under your shoulders.
2. Walk yourself under the bar so that you can set the bar behind your neck on your shoulders, then grip the bar with your hands facing forward.
3. Once the bar is set on your shoulders, slowly walk yourself at least 4 to 5 feet (1.21-1.52 m) away from the rack.
4. Stand with your feet about hip-width apart and knees slightly bent (*a*).
5. Keep your spine long and chin tucked as you hinge at your hips, moving them back behind you, making sure to keep your knees unlocked but not to bend them more (*b*).
6. Go only as far as you can while keeping your core engaged. Hold at the end range of motion for 1 to 2 seconds or for the desired amount of time.
7. Stand back up to your starting position, and complete the desired number of reps.

## Things to Keep in Mind

- Do not lock your knees. Make sure they are slightly bent for the whole exercise.
- Lower is not better with this movement. If your back starts to round, you lose engagement with your core.
- Attempt only the range of motion that feels good to you.
- Do not lean back or extend your lower back when you stand up.

## CONVENTIONAL OR AMERICAN DEADLIFT

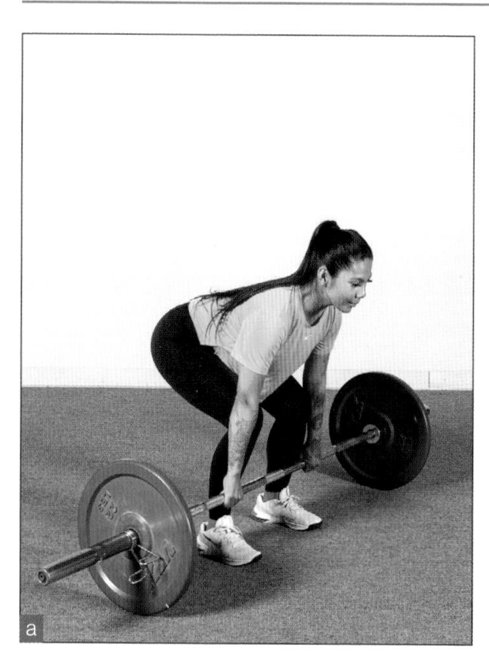
a

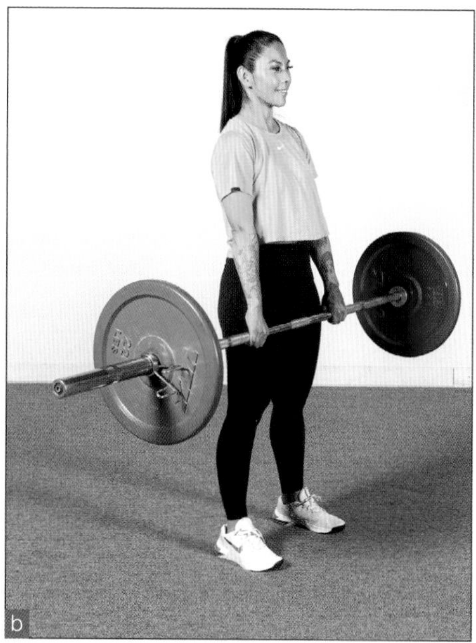
b

1. Set your barbell on the ground and stand behind it with your feet about hip-width apart.
2. Bend your knees and hinge at your hips, grabbing the bar with the grip that feels comfortable for you, with your arms outside of your knees.
3. Engage your core and pull your shoulders back as you push your feet into the ground to build tension (*a*).
4. Keep your core engaged as you stand up, picking the weight off the ground as you extend the knees (*b*).
5. If it is light enough, control the weight to put it back on the ground slowly. If you are on a lifting platform or proper flooring, you may release the weight at the top by simply letting the weight drop (note that some gyms may prohibit dropping weights).

### Things to Keep in Mind

- Occasional rounding of the back can happen in a conventional or American deadlift, but you should pick up the weight with your core and back engaged. Lifting a too-heavy weight with poor form for the sake of making a PR can lead to injuries.
- Make sure you are pushing the floor away from you with your feet as you stand up.

## Variations

### Sumo Conventional Deadlift

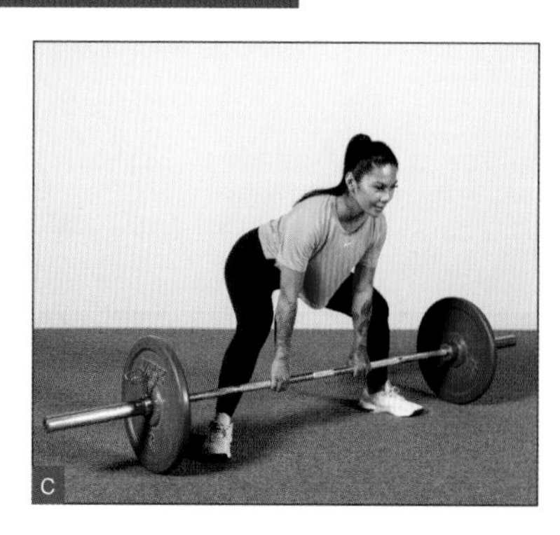
c

1. Set with your barbell on the ground and stand behind it with your feet wide and toes turned out.
2. Repeat steps 2 through 5 of the conventional or American deadlift (*c*).

### Staggered Conventional Deadlift

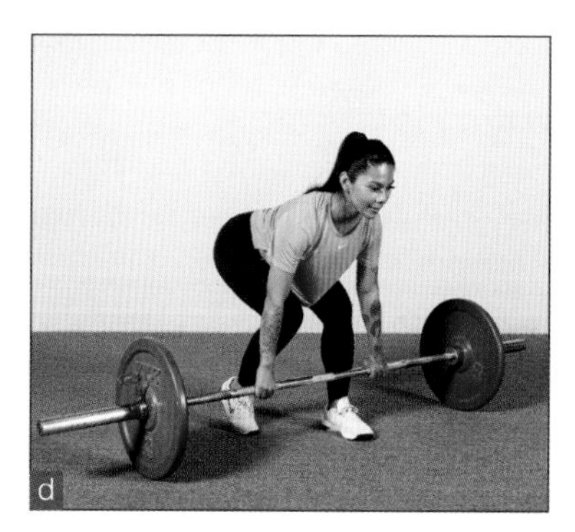
d

1. Set with your barbell on the ground and stand behind it with one foot about 6 inches (15.24 cm) behind the other with the heel lifted, but still hip-width apart.
2. Repeat steps 2 through 5 of the conventional or American deadlift (*d*).
3. Complete desired number of reps, then repeat on the other side.

## PRONATED, SUPINATED, AND MIXED GRIPS

When performing a conventional or American deadlift, you are typically lifting significantly heavier weight than you would with a Romanian deadlift. Varying your grip can help make the lift more comfortable for you. There is no right or wrong way to do it; I just want you to do what helps you execute the lift with good form.

The pronated or overhand grip (*a*) is the typical grip used with the American deadlift, but if you are a newer lifter, it may be a little more difficult to attain the core activation needed when doing the lift, so experimenting with either the supinated or mixed grip is a good option.

By using a supinated or underhand grip (*b*), some lifters are able to open their chest more, making it easier to squeeze their shoulder blades back so that they can focus on activating their core. I sometimes suggest this grip for those who are learning the deadlift.

In the mixed grip (*c*), you place one hand in an underhand (supinated) grip and one in an overhand (pronated) grip. Some people find this more comfortable than placing both hands in a pronated grip, and some even report that they feel stronger with this grip than with either a pronated or supinated grip.

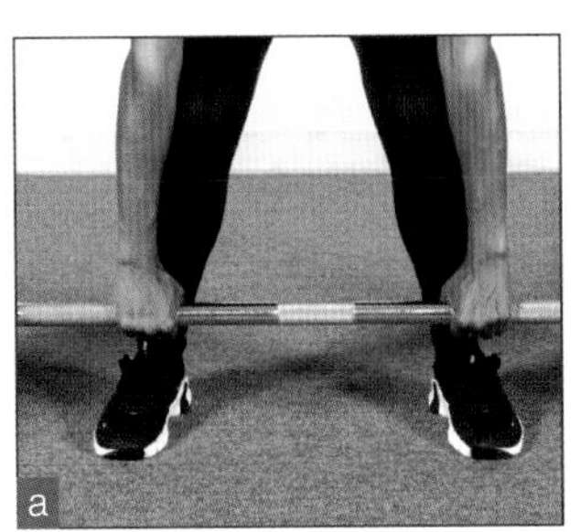
a

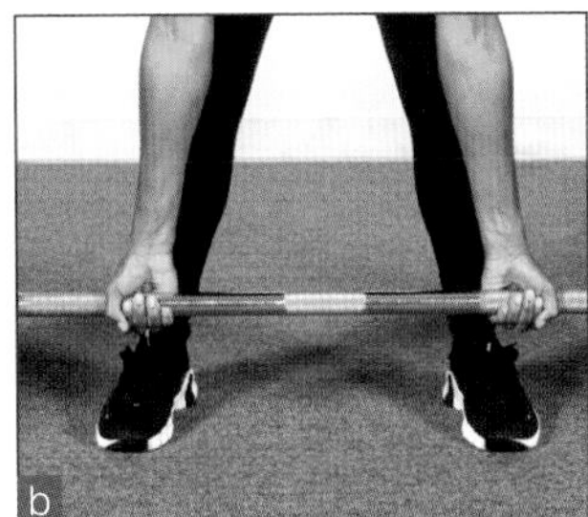
b

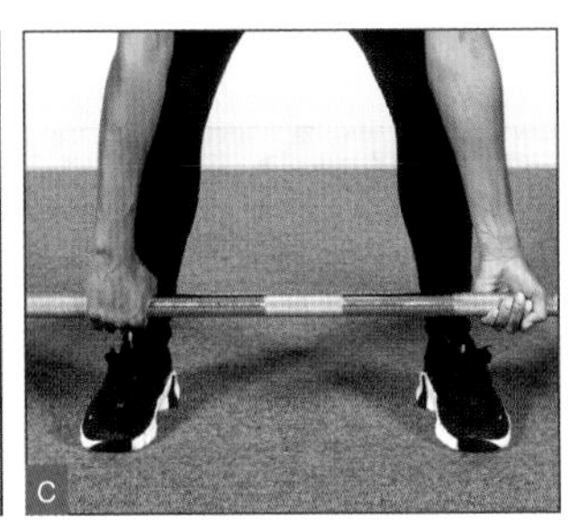
c

# SIDE-LYING HIP CIRCLES

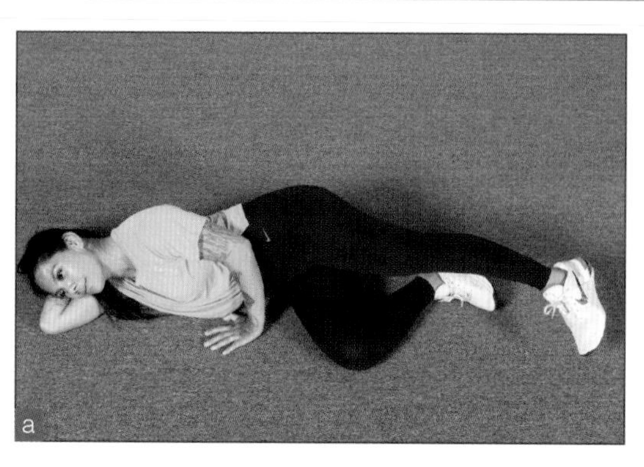
a

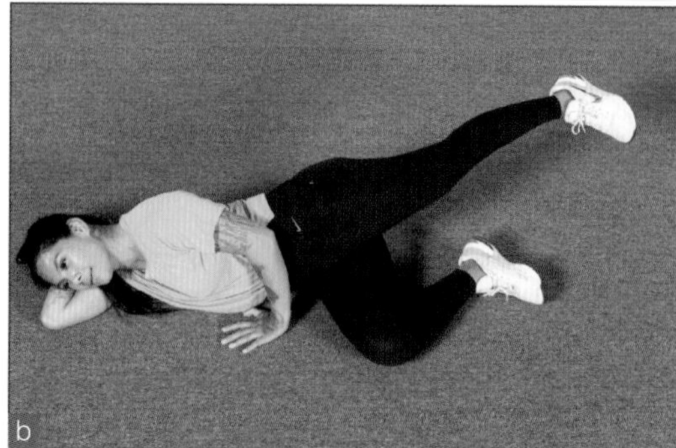
b

1. Lie on your side with your legs extended and hips stacked. Prop yourself up with your hand or your forearm (*a*).
2. Keep your rib cage in and still as you extend your top leg back and behind you, toes pointed down toward the floor.
3. Make a circle with the top leg as you move it around to the front of your body, bringing the leg back to the starting position (*b*).
4. Complete the desired number of reps, then repeat, going in the other direction.
5. Repeat with the other leg.

## Things to Keep in Mind

- Make sure you rotate your thighs with your toes pointed toward the ground to get the most out of the movement.
- As you get tired, avoid using your lower back by making sure you keep your core engaged to use your hip.

# SIDE-LYING ABDUCTION

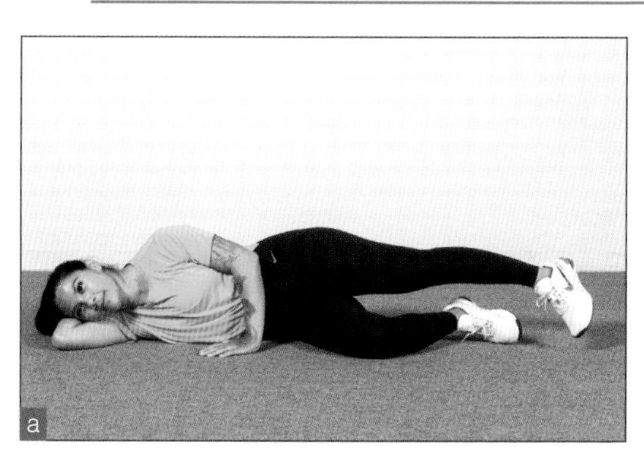

a

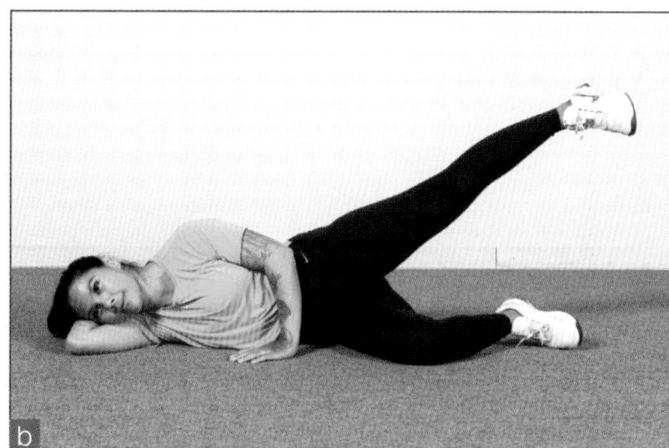

b

1. Lie on your side with your legs extended and hips stacked. Prop yourself up with your hand or your forearm.
2. Keep your rib cage in and rotate your top leg, turning your toes toward the ground (*a*).
3. Keep the rotation as you lift your top leg toward the sky (*b*).
4. Lower your leg back to the starting position.
5. Complete the desired number of reps, then repeat on the other side.

## Things to Keep in Mind

- Make sure you rotate your thighs so your toe points toward the ground to get the most out of the movement.
- As you get tired, you may start to use your lower back, so make sure you are keeping your core engaged to use your hips rather than your back.

# CABLE KICKBACK

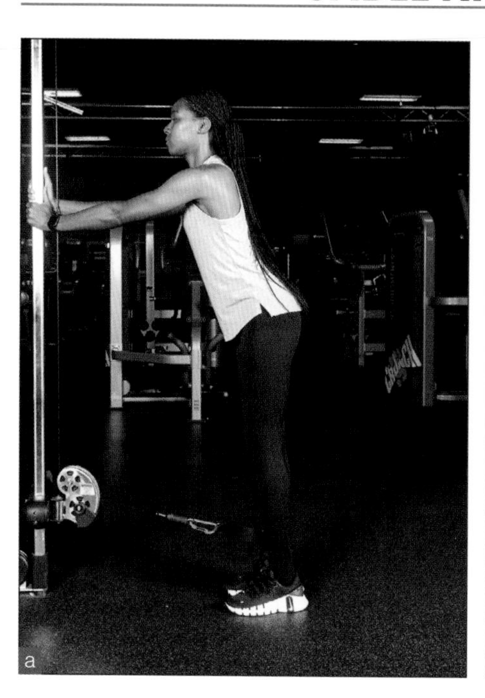

a

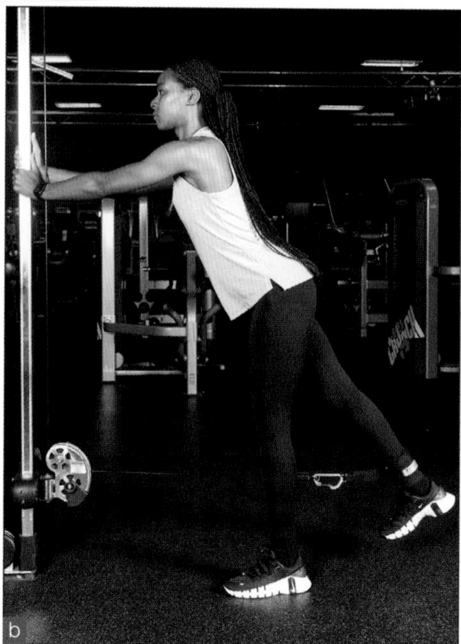

b

1. Wrap an ankle strap around your ankle and hook it to the cable machine.
2. Stand facing the anchor of the cable machine and walk yourself back a few steps to where you can feel a little tension in the cable.
3. Stand on the leg that does not have the ankle strap, with a soft bend in your knee (*a*).
4. If needed, hold onto the cable machine for extra stability.
5. Lift the leg with the ankle strap back and behind you, squeezing the glute, while keeping your spine long and core strong (*b*).
6. Slowly lower your leg back to the starting position and complete the desired number of reps.
7. Repeat with the other leg.

## Things to Keep in Mind

- You can stand on a small box or plate to give you more range of motion if it feels more comfortable.
- Make sure you are not arching your lower back as you kick the weight back; keep your core engaged and your pelvis tucked.

# CABLE ABDUCTION

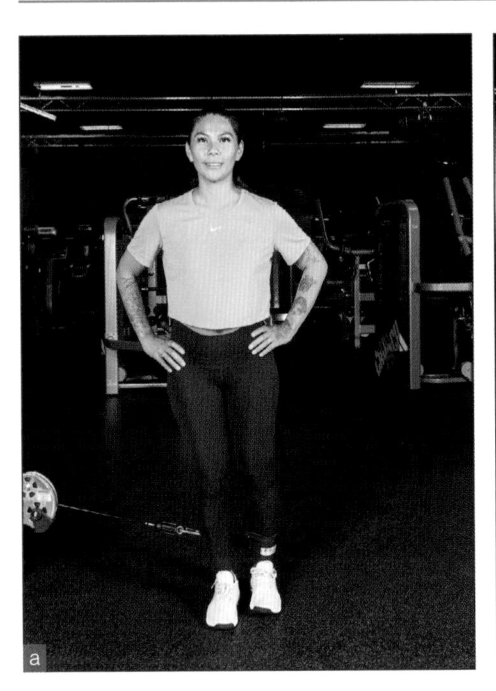

a

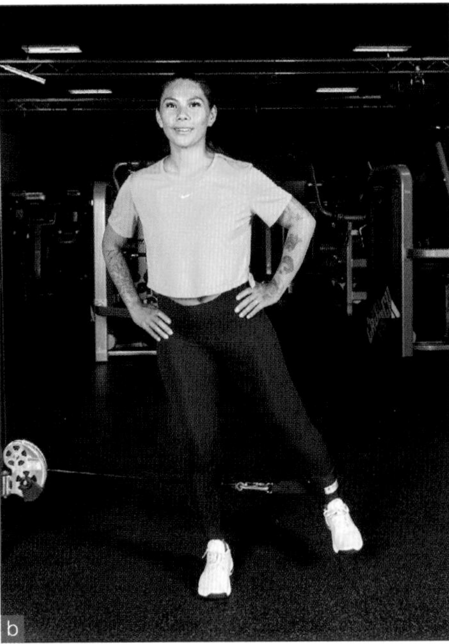

b

1. Wrap an ankle strap around your ankle and hook it to the cable machine.
2. Stand so that you are perpendicular (with your side to the anchor) and the ankle with the ankle strap is farther away from the anchor than the other ankle; there should be a little tension on the cable.
3. Stand on the leg that does not have the ankle strap, with a soft bend in your knee (*a*).
4. If needed, hold onto the cable machine for extra stability.
5. Lift the leg with the ankle strap away from your body to the side, leading with your heel, squeezing the glute, making sure to not lean too far in the other direction (*b*).
6. Slowly lower your leg back to the starting position and complete the desired number of reps.

## Things to Keep in Mind

- You can stand on a small box or plate to give you more range of motion if it feels more comfortable.

# CABLE ADDUCTION

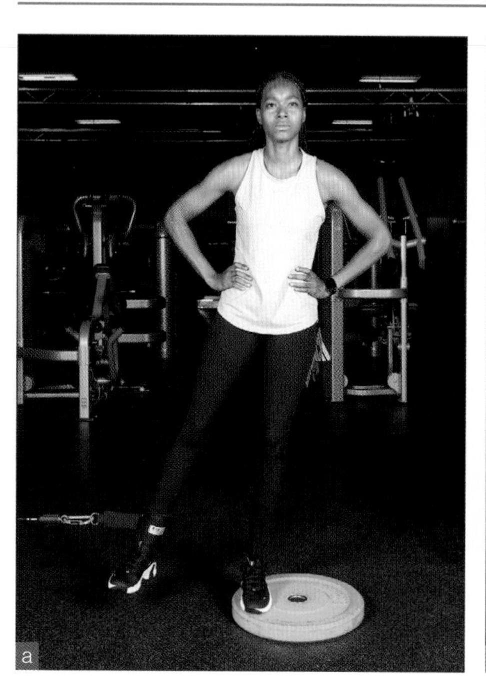
a

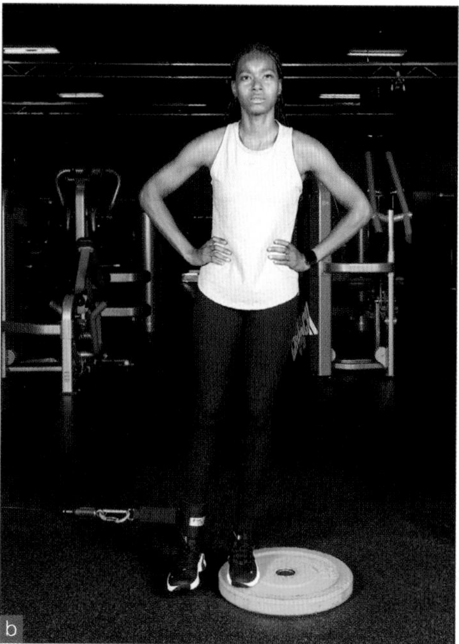
b

1. Wrap an ankle strap around your ankle and hook it to the cable machine
2. Stand so that you are perpendicular (with your side to the anchor) and the ankle with the ankle strap is closer to the anchor than the other ankle.
3. Stand on the leg that does not have the ankle strap with a soft bend in your knee and the other leg extended out to the side (*a*).
4. If needed, hold onto the cable machine for extra stability.
5. Move the leg with the ankle strap closer to your standing leg, keeping your spine long and core engaged (*b*).
6. Slowly bring your leg back out to the side to the starting position and complete the desired number of reps.
7. Repeat with the other leg.

## Things to Keep in Mind

- You can stand on a small box or plate to give you more range of motion if it feels more comfortable (see photos).

# 7

# HORIZONTAL AND VERTICAL PUSH

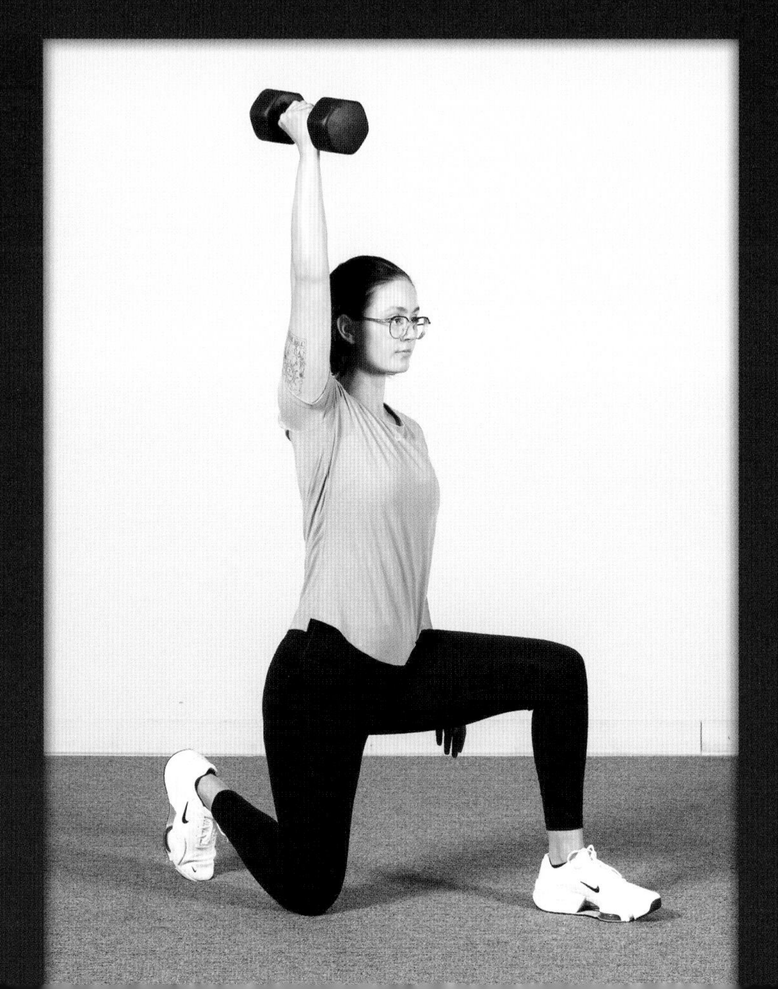

I like to categorize upper-body exercises by the two main motions: pushing and pulling. In this chapter, we focus on two categories of push movements in multiple planes of motion: vertical pushes and horizontal pushes. "Horizontal" and "vertical" refer to the direction you move the weight in relation to your body position. Push exercises include some of the more obvious ones, like push-ups, shoulder press, and chest press, but also include triceps extension, chest fly, and lateral raises. The dominant muscles worked in upper-body pushing movements are typically those in your chest, triceps, and shoulders.

Many of these exercises are done with dumbbells or cables and can be done by moving both arms at the same time or by alternating, one arm at a time. (If an exercise is meant to be alternating, this will be noted in the programs in part III.) Also, don't forget that it is always recommended to have a spotter when you are pushing a challenging weight.

**! *It is always recommended to have a spotter when pushing a challenging weight.***

## ELEVATED OR WALL PUSH-UP

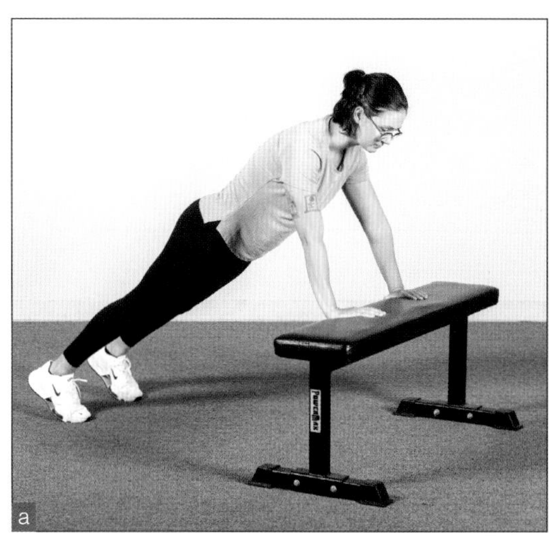
a

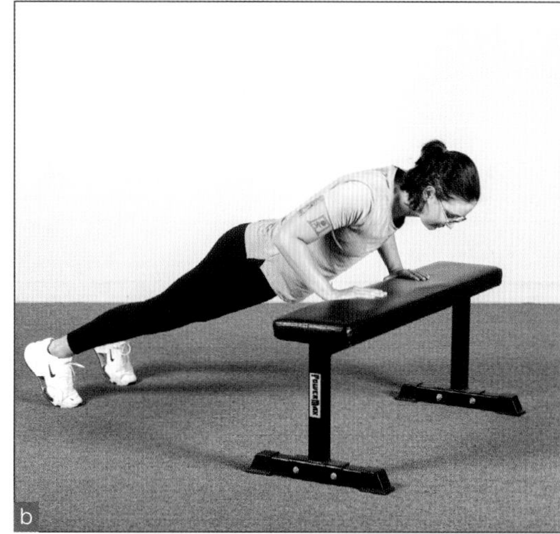
b

1. Place your hands on a wall or a sturdy elevated surface, like a box or bench.
2. Once you feel sturdy enough, walk your feet out so that you are in a straight line, adjusting your arm position if necessary to align with your armpits.
3. Tuck your pelvis and activate your core, so you are in a straight line as you press your hands into the wall or surface (*a*).
4. Bend your elbows as you bring your body closer to the surface in one line, going as low as you can while keeping your core engaged. Your hands should be in line with your armpits (*b*).
5. Extend your arms, pushing yourself away from the surface or wall, and repeat for the desired amount of reps

# DUMBBELL CHEST PRESS

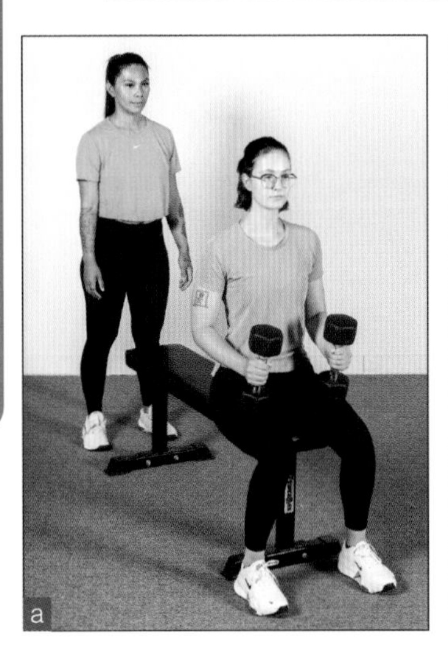
a

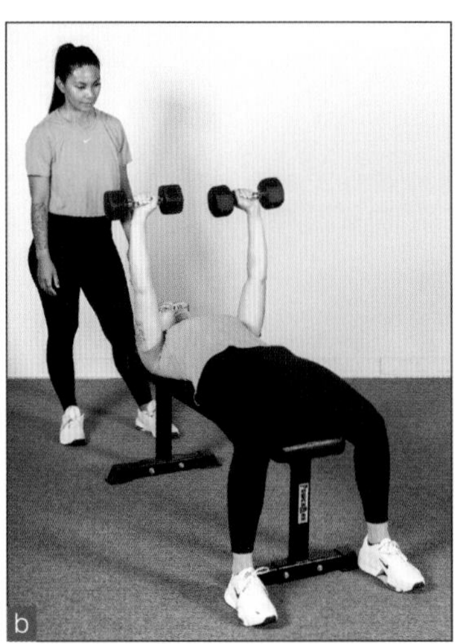
b

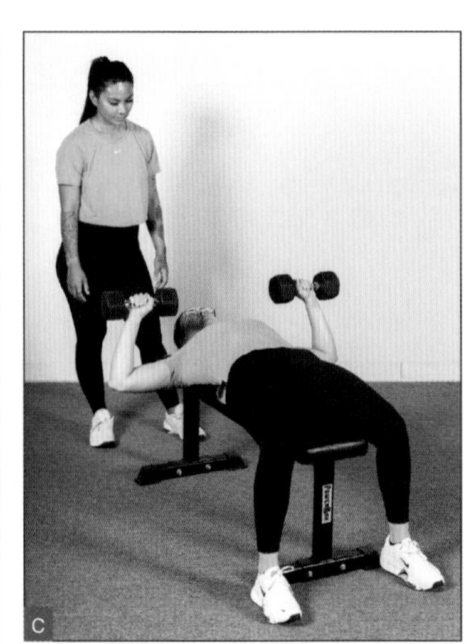
c

1. Sit at the end of a bench with a dumbbell on each thigh.
2. Gripping the dumbbells tight with your elbows hugged to your rib cage, slowly lie back on the bench, using your abs to keep the dumbbells close to your body as you lie back.
3. Press your feet into the ground to stabilize yourself as you bring the dumbbells in line with your chest, keeping your elbows bent (*a*).
4. Press the dumbbells up toward the ceiling, extending your arms straight and keeping your glutes and abs engaged (*b*).
5. Slowly, with control, lower the dumbbells back to the starting position and complete the desired number of reps (*c*).
6. When finished, slowly lower the dumbbells to the ground safely or hug your elbows back into your chest to return to the seated starting position.

## Things to Keep in Mind

- Push your feet into the ground to help you press the dumbbells up.
- Exhale as you press the dumbbells up.
- I recommend having a spotter for this exercise.

## Variation

- This exercise can also be done by alternating one arm at a time.

# BARBELL CHEST PRESS

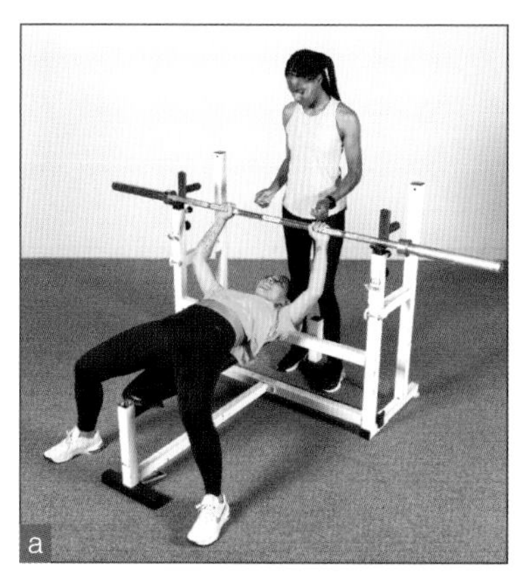
a

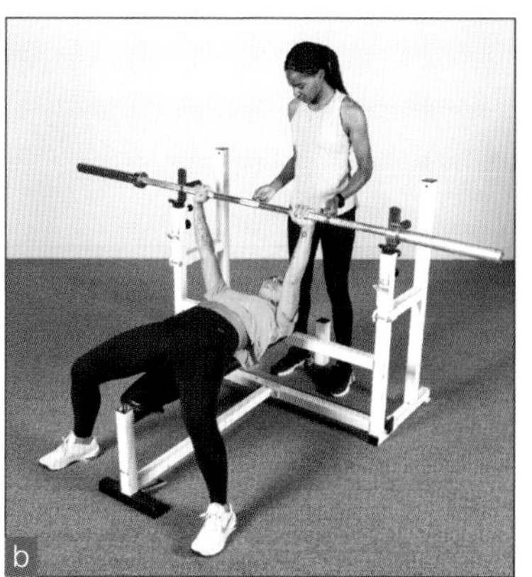
b

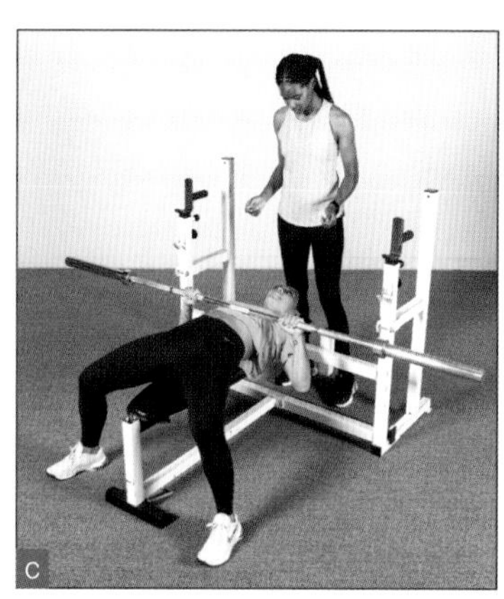
c

1. Lie on a bench with a weight rack overhead. The rack should be positioned so that the height of the pins where the bar is held allows your elbows to be bent at about 90 degrees. The bar should be lined up with your armpits.
2. Lie with your knees bent and your feet on the floor.
3. Press your feet into the ground to stabilize yourself as you place your hands on the bar with an overhand grip about shoulder-width apart (*a*).
4. Press the bar away from the pins on the rack, extending your arms completely (*b*).
5. Restabilize yourself, pressing your heels into the ground again while contracting your glutes and abs.
6. Keeping that tension, slowly lower the bar down in line with your chest, bending your elbows, letting the bar touch your sternum (*c*).
7. Keeping the same tension, press the weight back up, extending your arms. This is one rep.
8. Complete the desired number of reps.
9. When finished, keep your arms extended and shift the weight back to rerack the weight. Your spotter can help you guide it back to the pins.

## Things to Keep in Mind

- If you are new to this exercise, practice with a lighter or empty bar (bar without weight) to make sure you have your setup correct.
- Push your feet into the ground on the way up to help you lift.
- Exhale as you press the bar up.
- I recommend having a spotter for this exercise.

# DUMBBELL FLOOR PRESS

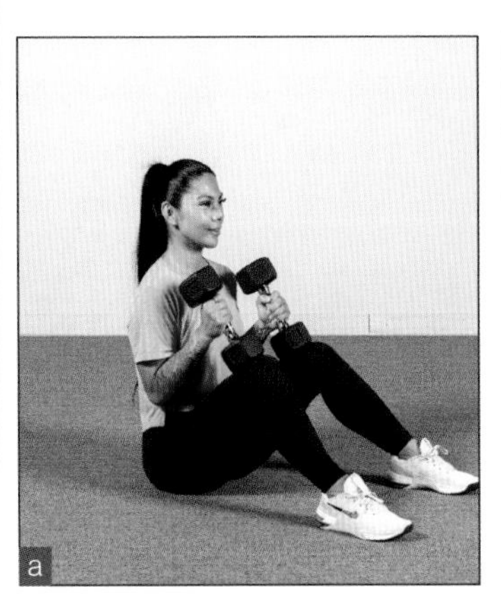
a

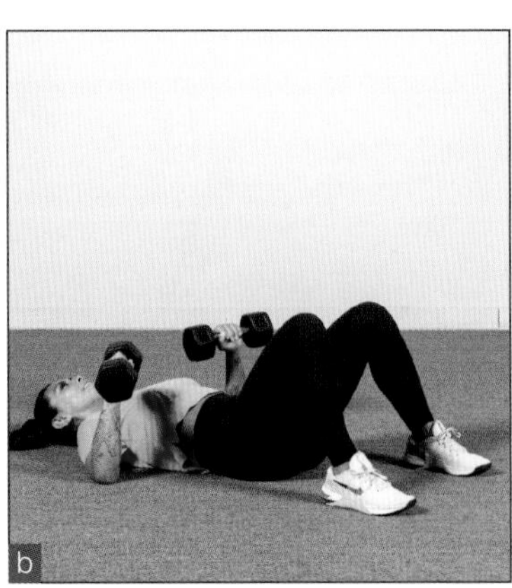
b

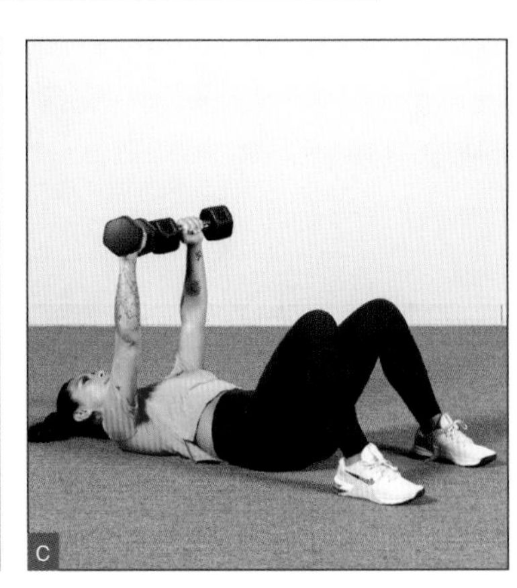
c

1. Start seated on the floor with your dumbbells on your thighs (*a*).
2. Gripping your dumbbells tight with your elbows hugged to your rib cage, slowly lie back on the floor, using your abs to keep your dumbbells close to your body as you lie back.
3. Bend your knees so your heels are about 12 inches (30.48 cm) away from your butt (*b*).
4. Press your dumbbells above your chest, up toward the ceiling keeping your arms straight (*c*).
5. Slowly, with control, lower the dumbbells so that your elbows bend all the way down to the ground, about 45 degrees away from your body.
6. Press the dumbbells back up toward the sky. That is one rep.
7. Complete the desired number of reps.
8. When finished, slowly lower your dumbbells down to the ground safely or hug your elbows into your chest to reverse back to the seated starting position.

## Things to Keep in Mind

- You will not get a full range of motion on this movement the way you would on a bench, so you may be able to use a heavier weight than usual.

## Variation

- This exercise can also be done by alternating one arm at a time.

# CABLE CHEST PRESS

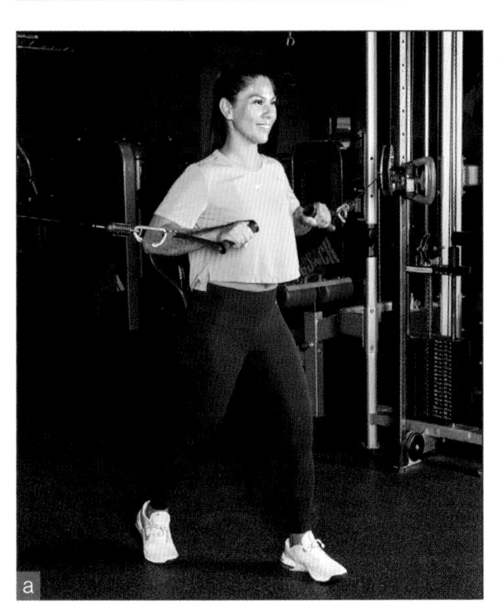


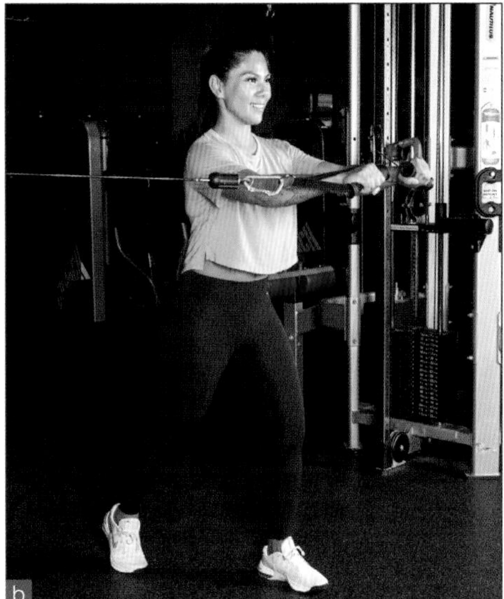


1. Adjust the settings on the double cable machine so that your arms are in line just under your chest.
2. Standing in the middle of the two anchors, stand with one foot in front of the other and grasp a handle in each hand.
3. Walk yourself 2 to 3 inches (5.08-7.62 cm) in front of the anchors so that there is tension on the cables, with your hands in line next to your chest with your elbows bent behind you, and your palms facing toward the ground. This is your starting position (*a*).
4. Keeping your posture tall and your rib cage in, press the cable handles forward and away from you so that you are fully extending your arms (*b*).
5. Hold briefly, then slowly return to resting position. Complete the desired number of reps.

## Things to Keep in Mind

- You may need to adjust yourself a few times to make sure the cable feels right and isn't catching on your arms.

## Variation

- This exercise can also be done by alternating one arm at a time.

# DUMBBELL CHEST FLY

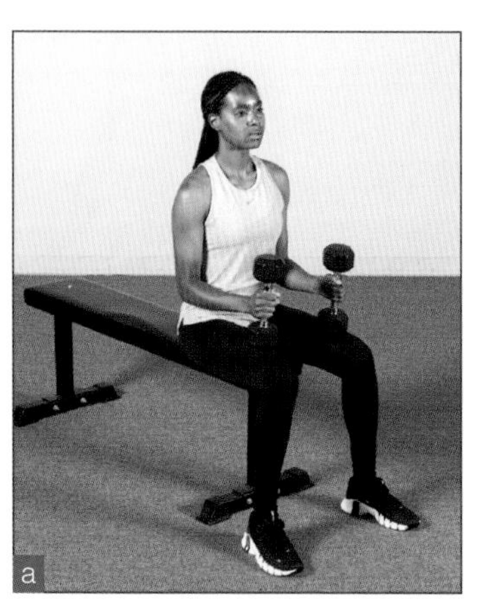


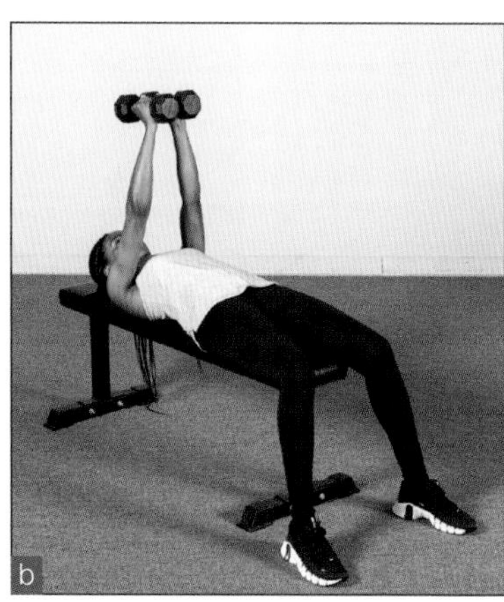


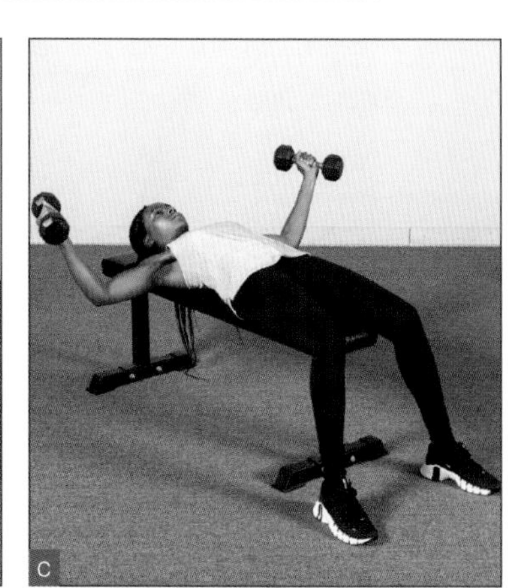


1. Sit at the end of a weight bench, holding the dumbbells on your thighs (*a*).
2. Gripping the dumbbells tight, with your elbows hugged to your rib cage, slowly lie back onto the bench, using your abs to keep the dumbbells close to your body as you lie back.
3. With your palms facing each other, press your dumbbells up toward the sky with your elbows slightly bent. This is your starting position (*b*).
4. Keeping the same bend in your elbow, lower the dumbbells out to the side, in line with your chest or as far as you comfortably can (*c*).
5. Slowly bring your dumbbells back to the starting position, and complete the desired number of reps.

## Things to Keep in Mind

- Make sure the movement is coming from your shoulders and not your elbows. Imagine a hinge in your shoulders rather than a bend in your elbows.
- Make sure your arms are in line with your chest when you lower them down to the side. Attempt only a range of motion that feels comfortable.

## Variation

- This exercise can also be done by alternating one arm at a time.

## CABLE CHEST FLY

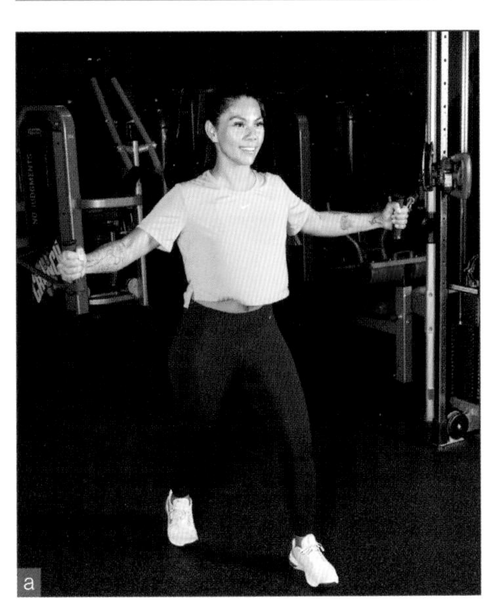
a

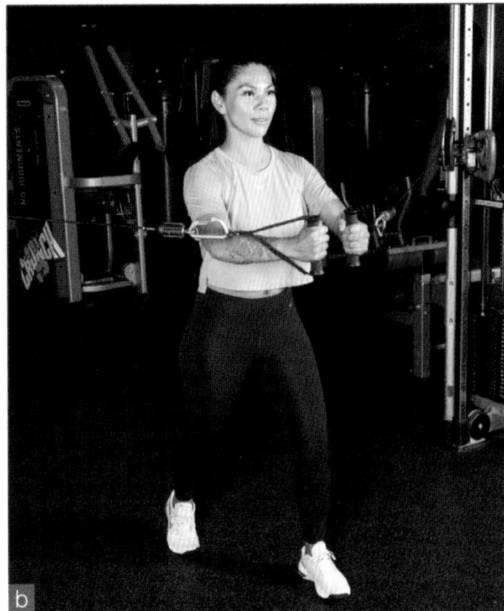
b

1. Adjust the double cable machine so that your arms are in line just under your chest.
2. Standing in the middle of the two anchors, stand with one foot in front of the other and grasp a handle in each hand.
3. Walk yourself 2 to 3 inches (5.08-7.62 cm) in front of the anchors so that there is tension on the cables, with your arms extended in line with your chest and a soft bend in your elbows. This is your starting position (*a*).
4. Keeping the same bend in your elbows and holding your rib cage in, slowly bring the handles closer together, as if you were hugging a giant ball in front of you (*b*).
5. Hold briefly, then slowly return to the starting position. Complete the desired number of reps.

### Things to Keep in Mind

- Make sure the movement is coming from your shoulders and not your elbows. Imagine a hinge in your shoulders rather than a bend in your elbows.

### Variation

- This exercise can also be done by alternating one arm at a time.

# HALF-KNEELING OVERHEAD PRESS

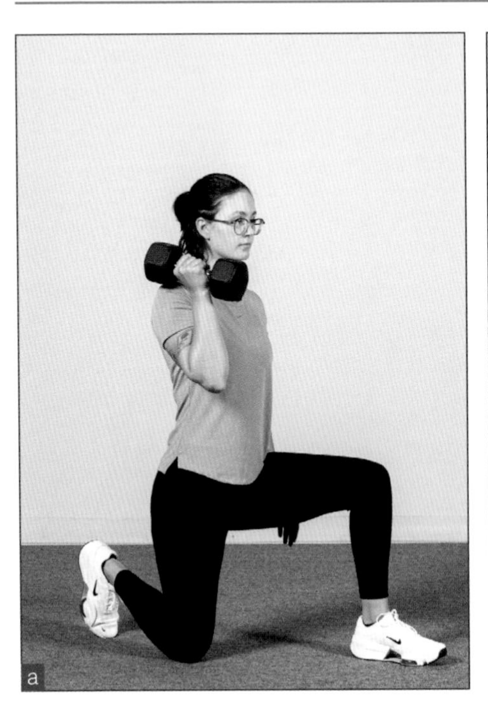
a

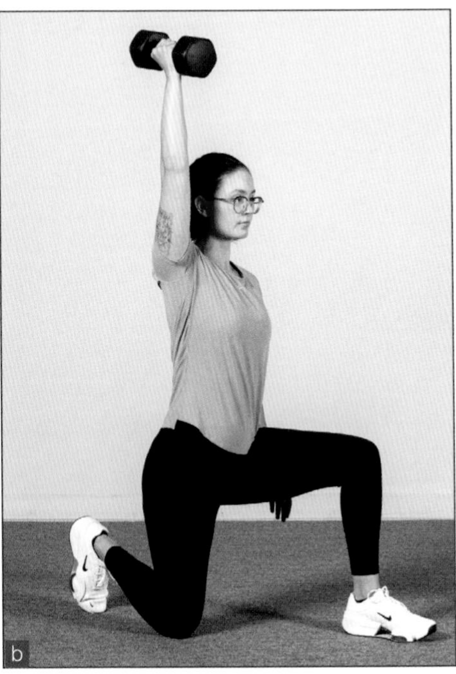
b

1. Start with your right knee on the ground and your left knee up so you are in a half-kneeling position. Make sure your stance isn't too narrow so that you are stable.
2. The toes of your right foot should be curled under so your foot is flexed. If your flexibility does not allow this, the top of your foot can be flat on the ground.
3. Hold one dumbbell in your right hand at your shoulder, in a neutral position, with your elbow hugged in toward your rib cage (*a*).
4. Keeping your pelvis tucked and rib cage in, press the dumbbell straight up toward the sky, straightening your arm all the way so that your biceps meets close to your ear (*b*).
5. Lower the dumbbell with control and complete the desired number of reps.
6. Repeat on the other side, making sure to switch your knees.

## Things to Keep in Mind

- Make sure the knee on the floor is the side that has the dumbbell.
- Keep your shoulders stacked over your rib cage and your rib cage stacked over your hips, with your pelvis tucked.

# TALL KNEELING OVERHEAD PRESS

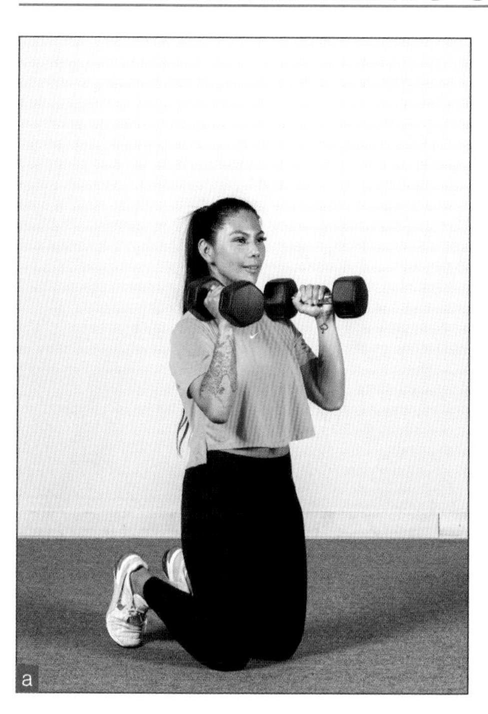
a

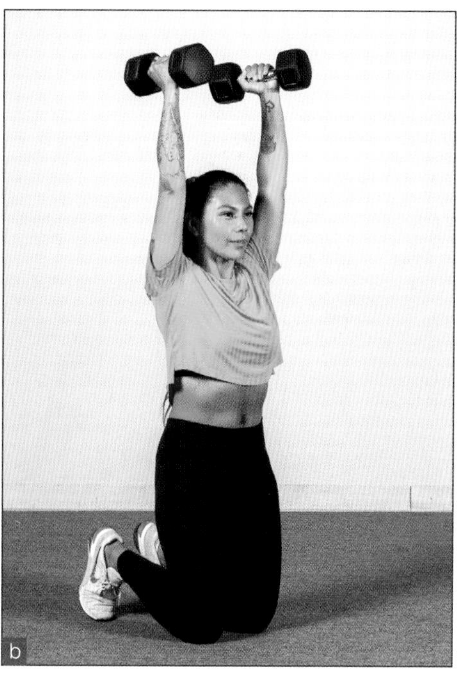
b

1. Start with both knees on the ground about hip-width apart, with your hips fully extended.
2. Your toes should be curled under, so that your feet are flexed. If your flexibility does not allow this, the top of your feet can be flat on the ground.
3. Hold one dumbbell in each hand at your shoulders, in a neutral position, with your elbows hugged in toward your rib cage (*a*).
4. Keeping your pelvis tucked and rib cage in, press your dumbbells straight up toward the sky, straightening your arms all the way so that your biceps meet your ears (*b*).
5. Lower the dumbbells with control and complete the desired number of reps.

## Things to Keep in Mind

- Keep your shoulders stacked over your rib cage, and your rib cage stacked over your hips, with your pelvis tucked.

## Variation

- This exercise can also be done by alternating one arm at a time.

# DUMBBELL OVERHEAD PRESS

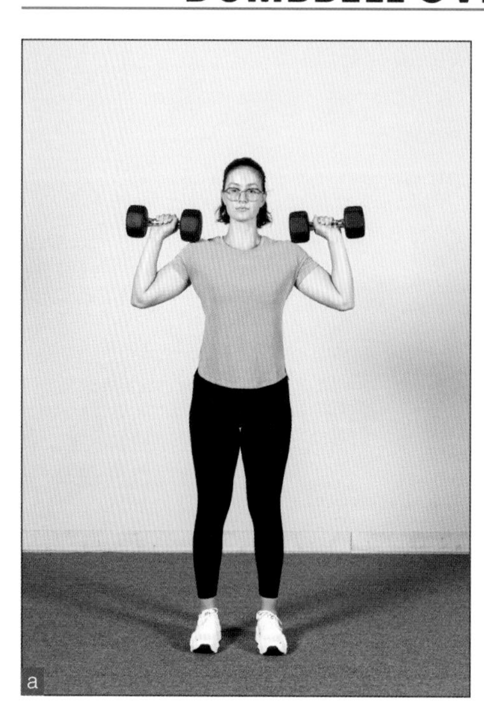
a

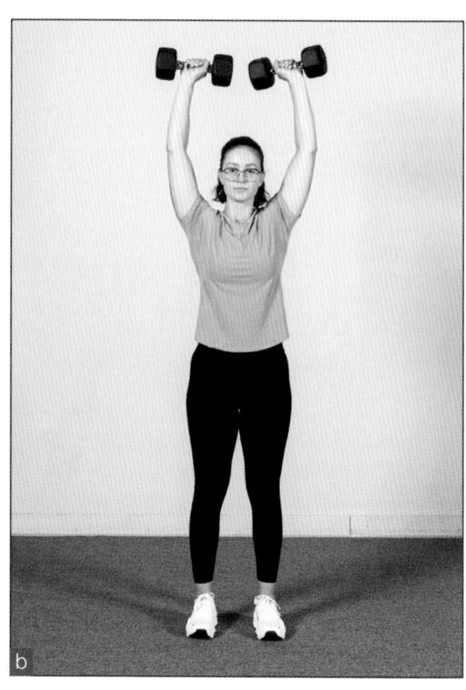
b

1. Stand with your feet hip-width apart and a dumbbell in each hand.
2. Bring your dumbbells up and in line with your shoulders with your elbows bent and your palms rotated away from you (*a*).
3. Keeping your rib cage in, press your dumbbells up and overhead, extending your arms completely, so that your biceps are in line with your ears (*b*).
4. Slowly, with control, lower the dumbbells back down, and complete the desired number of reps.

## Things to Keep in Mind

- Try not to use your legs to help press the dumbbells up.
- Keep your shoulders stacked over your rib cage, and your rib cage stacked over your hips, with your pelvis tucked.
- When trying a new heavy weight, a spotter may be needed.

## Variations

- This exercise can also be done by alternating one arm at a time.
- This exercise can be done in a staggered stance.

# DUMBBELL PUSH PRESS

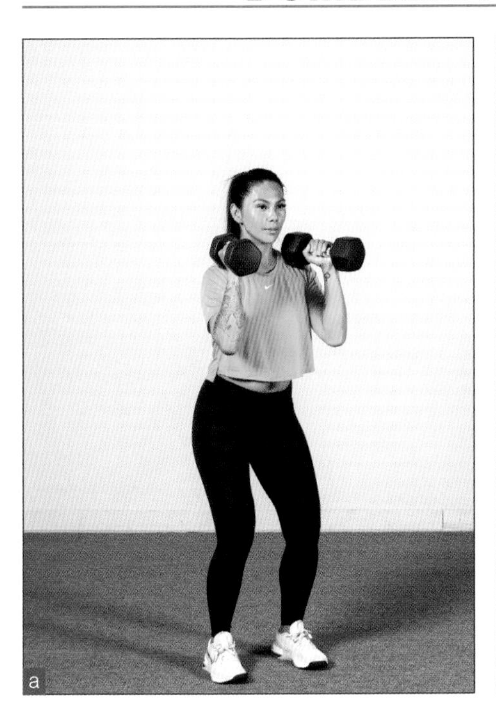

a

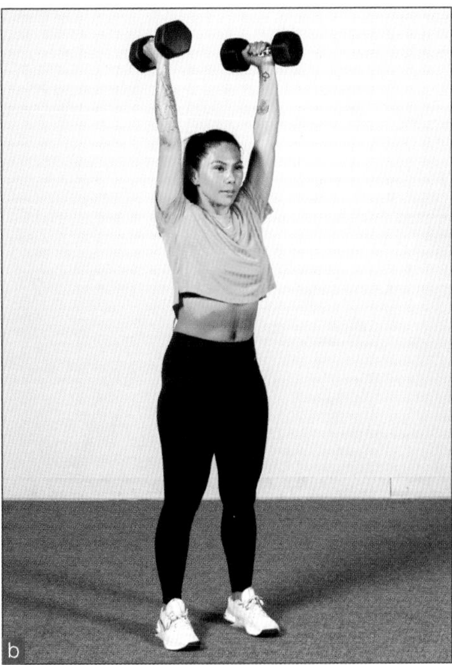

b

1. Stand with your feet hip-width apart with a dumbbell in each hand.
2. Bring your dumbbells up and in line with your shoulders with your elbows bent and your palms facing each other (*a*).
3. Bend your knees slightly to use the power from your legs to press your dumbbells up, extending your arms completely, so that your biceps are in line with your ears (*b*).
4. Slowly lower the dumbbells back down with control, and complete the desired number of reps.

## Things to Keep in Mind

- Keep your shoulders stacked over your rib cage, and your rib cage stacked over your hips, with your pelvis tucked.

## Variations

- This exercise can also be done by alternating one arm at a time.
- This exercise can be done in a staggered stance.

# DUMBBELL ARNOLD PRESS

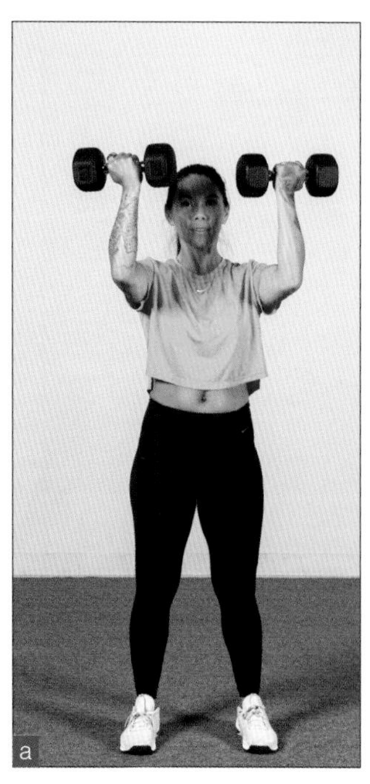

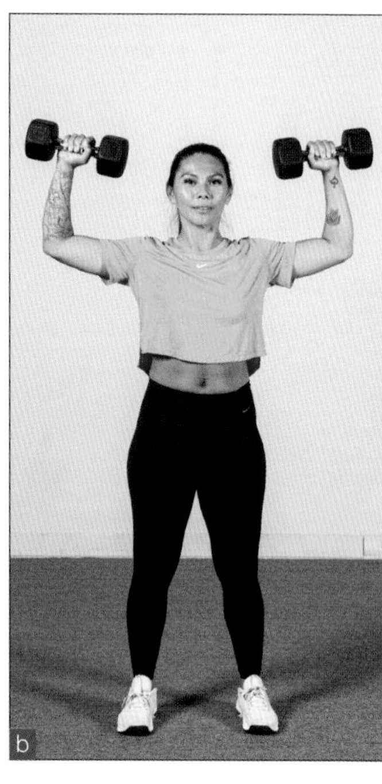

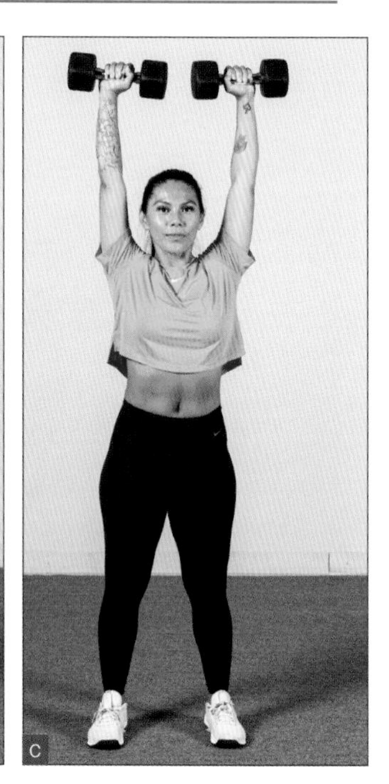

1. Stand with your feet hip-width apart and a dumbbell in each hand.
2. Bring your dumbbells up and in line with your shoulders with your elbows bent and your palms backward.
3. Lift your arms so that your elbows are in line with your shoulders, and your palms are facing you, creating two 90-degree angles. This is your starting position (*a*).
4. Open your arms out to the side so that your palms are facing away from you. While keeping your rib cage in, hold briefly. This is the second position (*b*).
5. Extend your arms overhead so that your arms are straight and your biceps are in line with your ears; hold briefly (*c*).
6. Slowly lower the dumbbells back down to the second position, and hold briefly.
7. Return to the starting position, and complete the desired number of reps.

## Things to Keep in Mind

- Do not rush this movement; it can be fluid, but make sure you hit each stopping point and keep your elbows high.
- Keep your shoulders stacked over your rib cage, and your rib cage stacked over your hips, with your pelvis tucked.
- When trying a heavy weight for the first time, a spotter may be needed.

## Variations

- This exercise can also be done by alternating one arm at a time.
- This exercise can be done in a seated position or in a staggered stance (one foot slightly in front of the other).

# DUMBBELL FRONT RAISE



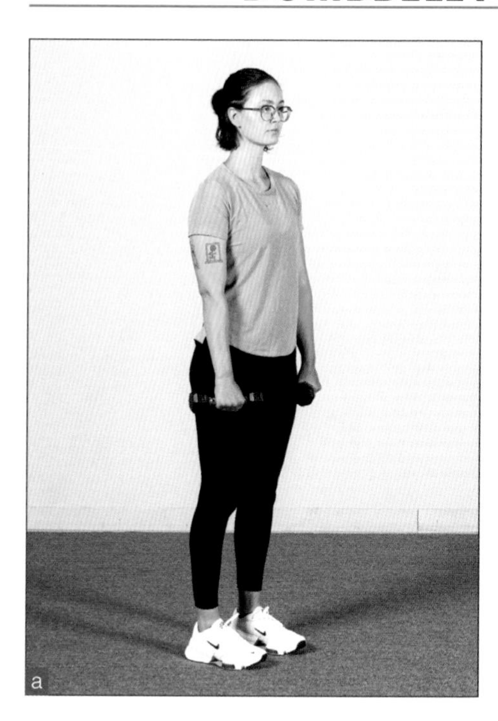


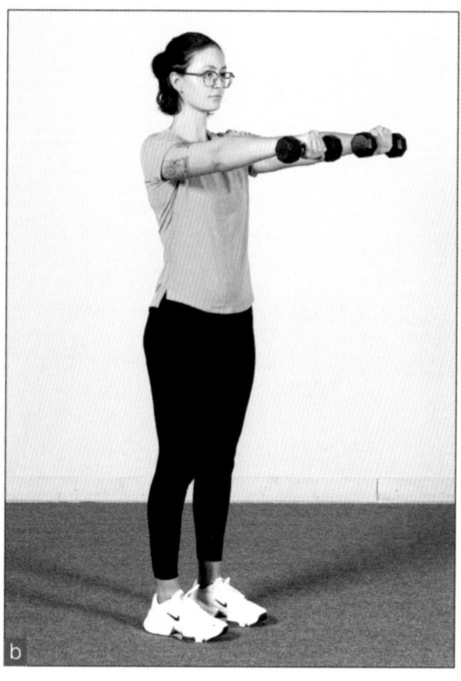


1. Stand with your feet hip-width apart. Hold a dumbbell in each hand in front of your thighs (*a*).
2. Lift your dumbbells forward, in line with your shoulders, with your arms extended as straight as you can, keeping your posture tall and not leaning back (*b*).
3. Hold briefly, then lower down with control.
4. Complete the desired number of reps.

## Things to Keep in Mind

- Do not swing the dumbbells up with momentum or lean back as you lift.
- If you are in between weight (i.e., one weight is too light and the next heaviest weight is too heavy), you can bend your elbows slightly.

## Variation

- This exercise can also be done by alternating one arm at a time.

# DUMBBELL LATERAL RAISE

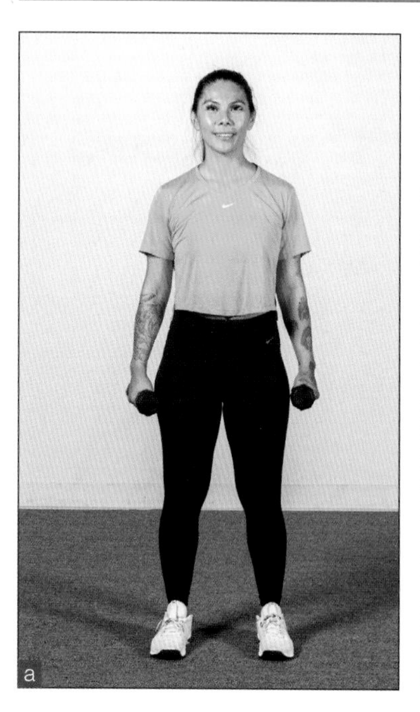

a

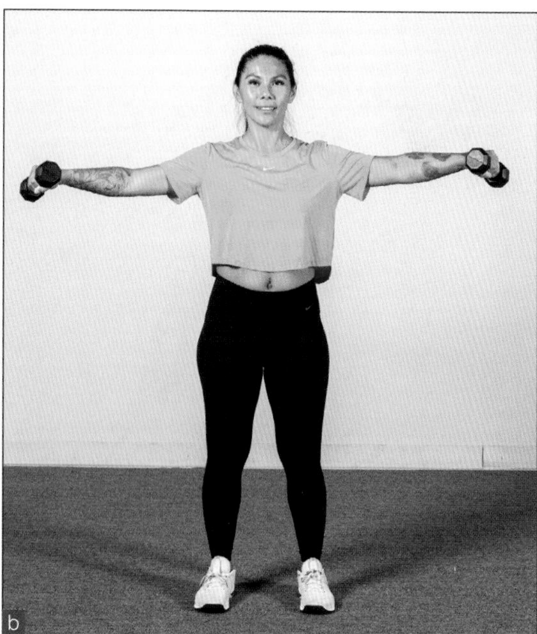

b

1. Stand with your feet hip-width apart and a dumbbell in each hand at your side (*a*).
2. Lift your dumbbells out to the side, in line with your shoulders, with your arms extended as straight as you can, keeping your posture tall and your rib cage in (*b*).
3. Hold briefly, then lower down with control.
4. Complete the desired number of reps.

## Things to Keep in Mind

- Do not swing your dumbbells with momentum as you lift them up.
- If you are in between weight, you can bend your elbows slightly.

## Variation

- This exercise can also be done by alternating one arm at a time.

# TRICEPS KICKBACK

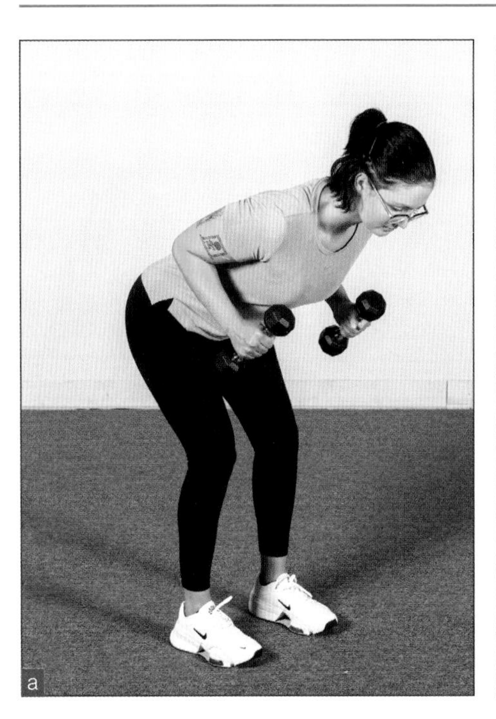

a

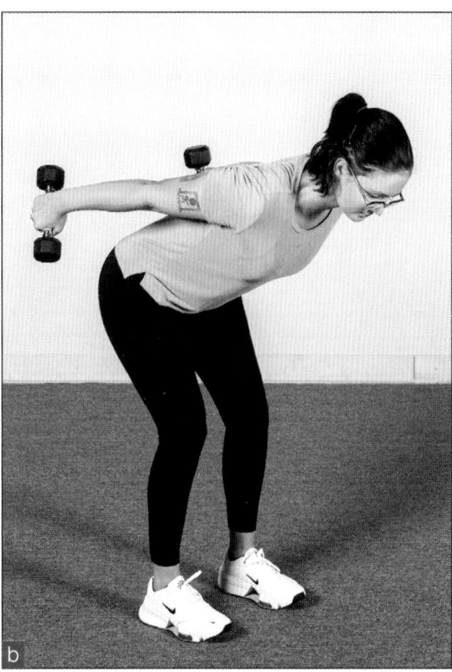

b

1. Stand with your feet hip-width apart and a dumbbell in each hand at your side.
2. Hinge at your hips, keeping your spine long, bending only to the lowest point at which you can keep your core engaged and your spine long.
3. Hold there, and bend your elbows so that the weights are near your shoulders. This is your starting position (*a*).
4. Keeping your shoulder blades squeezed together, hinge at your elbows. Using only your forearms, move the dumbbells back toward your hips, straightening your arms (*b*).
5. Hold for 1 to 2 seconds, then return to your starting position.
6. Complete the desired number of reps.

## Things to Keep in Mind

- Keep your elbows up higher than your back for the whole time.

## Variation

- This exercise can also be done by alternating one arm at a time.

# LYING TRICEPS EXTENSION

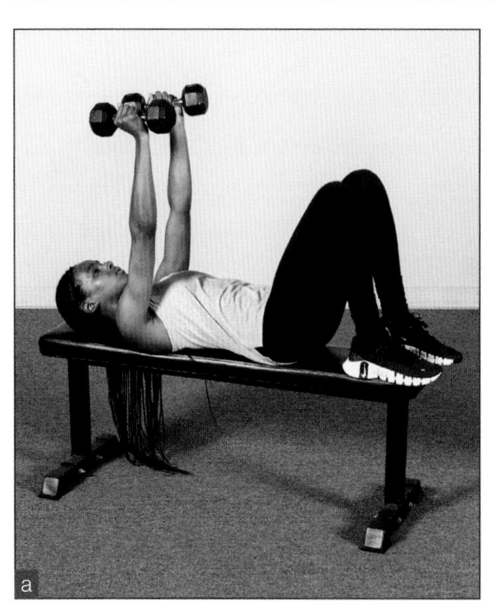
a

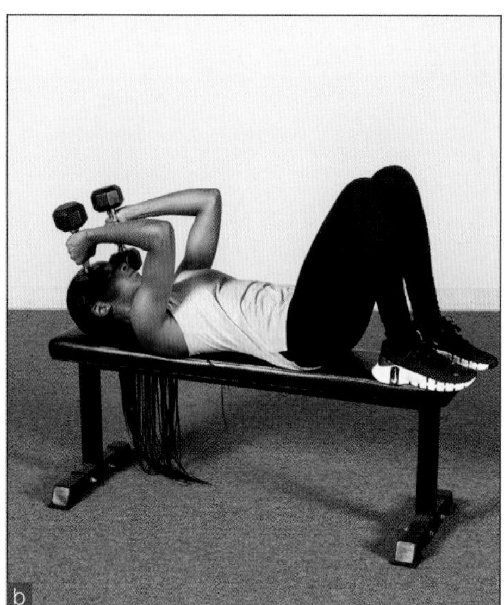
b

1. Sit at the end of a weight bench with a dumbbell in each hand.
2. Lie back with your feet on the floor (or you can place your feet on the bench with the knees bent) and arms extended above your chest with your palms facing each other (*a*).
3. Hinging at your elbows, move only your forearms to lower the dumbbells toward your temples, as if you were putting on sunglasses (*b*).
4. Slowly return the dumbbells to the starting position, and complete the desired number of reps.

## Things to Keep in Mind

- Make sure you move your forearms only by hinging at your elbows.

## Variation

- This exercise can also be done by alternating one arm at a time.

# 8

# HORIZONTAL AND VERTICAL PULL

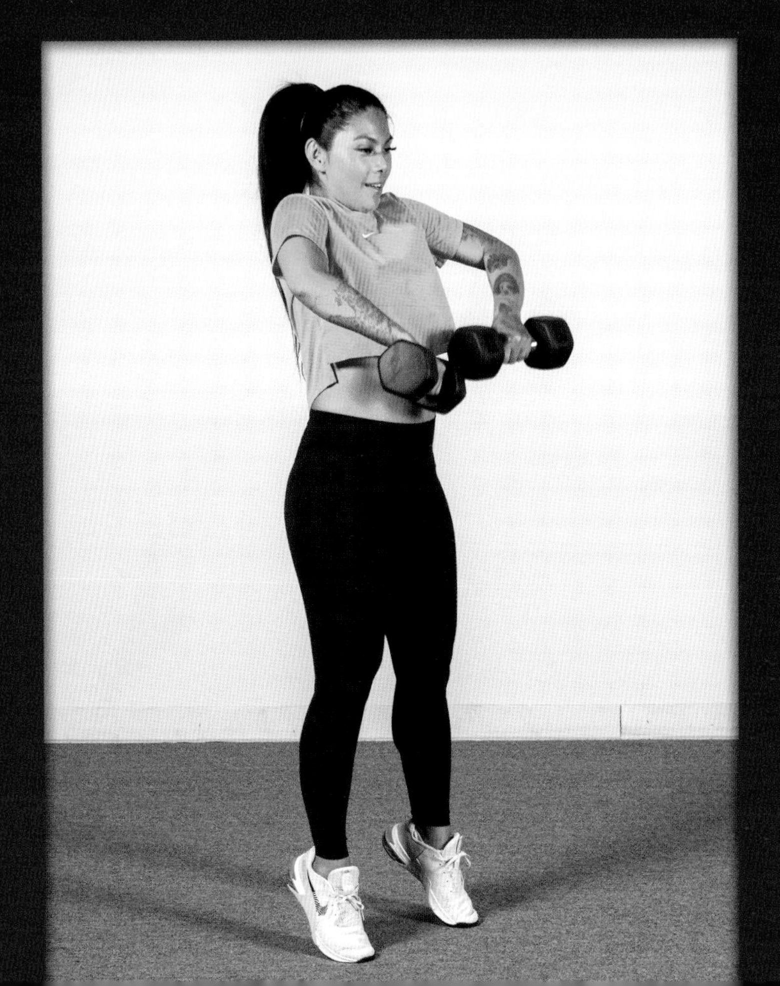

Upper-body pulling movements are at the top of my list for exercises that people need more of. Because most of us are constantly on our phones or computers, we tend to see a lot of rounding of the backs and shoulders with a forward head posture (see figure 8.1). The more we can strengthen our back muscles with pulling motions, the more we can help combat that forward head posture.

Many of the exercises that are done with dumbbells or cables can be done by moving both arms at the same time or by alternating one arm at a time. (If an exercise is meant to be alternating, this will be noted in the programs in part III.)

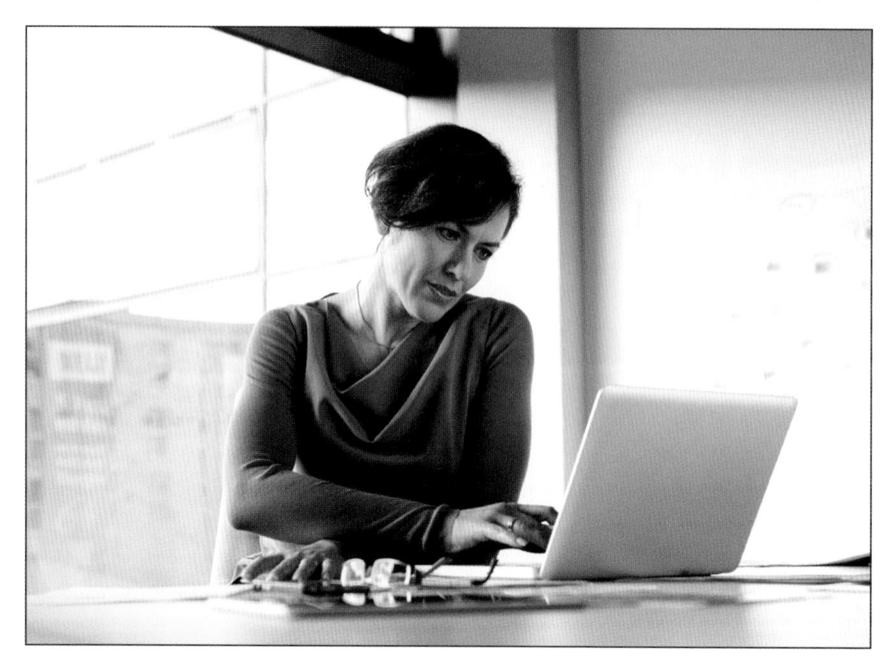

**FIGURE 8.1** Rounded posture in the back and shoulders is common for someone sitting at a desk for extended periods.
Westend61/Getty Images

# INVERTED ROW

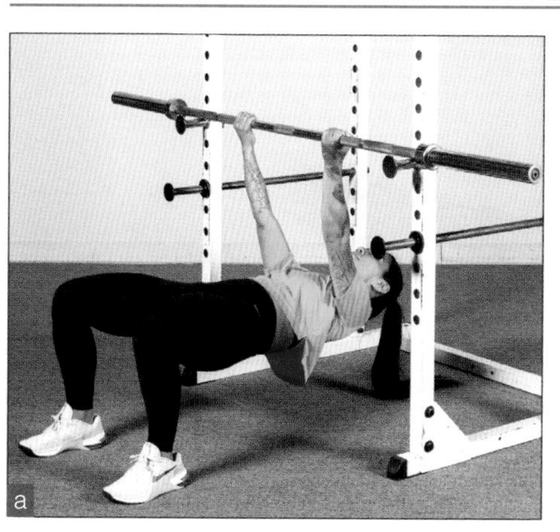
a

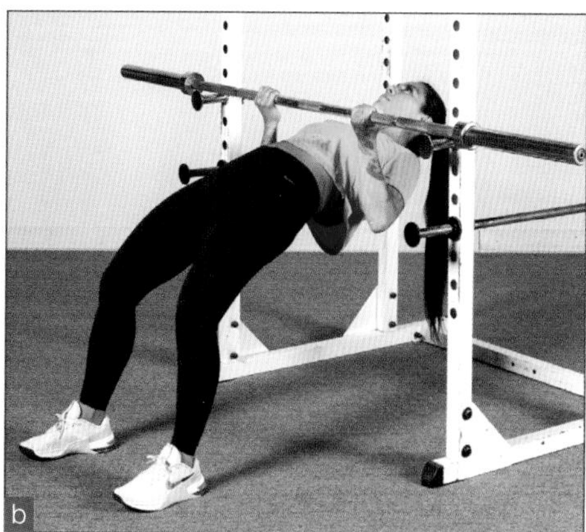
b

1. Bring a barbell or Smith machine bar to a low position, about in line with your hips. The lower the bar is, the more challenging it will be, but you also don't want it to be so low that you will not be able to extend your arms completely. You may need to adjust the height.
2. Get down on the floor and position yourself under the bar. Placing your hands about shoulder-width apart, grip the bar with an overhand or underhand grip (whichever is indicated in workout programs in part III).
3. Walk your feet out so that your chest is under the bar and your body is straight. You can bend your knees to a 90-degree angle or you can straighten your legs, with your feet flexed and heels on the ground. (A bend in the knees makes it easier.) This is your starting position (*a*).
4. Pull your chest to the bar, driving your elbows back and squeezing your shoulder blades together (*b*).
5. Hold for 1 to 2 seconds, and then slowly lower yourself back down into the starting position. Complete the desired number of reps.

## Things to Keep in Mind

- Ensure that the bar is stable so it doesn't move as you pull yourself up.
- Make sure you align yourself so that the bar is above your chest when your arms are extended.
- When you pull yourself to the bar, make sure your hands are in line with your chest, not your stomach.

## INTERCHANGING DUMBBELLS WITH BARBELLS

Some of the following exercises can be done with dumbbells or barbells, as long as both arms are moving at the same time. There may be a shift in the grip with dumbbells versus a barbell. For example, when you do a bent-over row with dumbbells, the grip looks more like a neutral grip, with your palms facing each other. When you hold a barbell, the grip is either pronated (overhand) or supinated (underhand). The general motion is the same, but different (smaller) muscles may be emphasized as the grip varies. Still, the prime movers remain the same. Each workout specifies which piece of equipment you will use, along with the grip. If the designated piece of equipment isn't available, you can use what is at hand.

# DUMBBELL BENT-OVER ROW

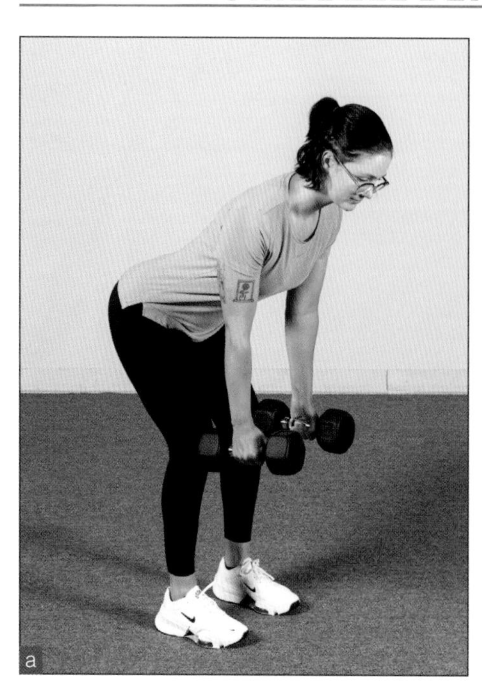
a

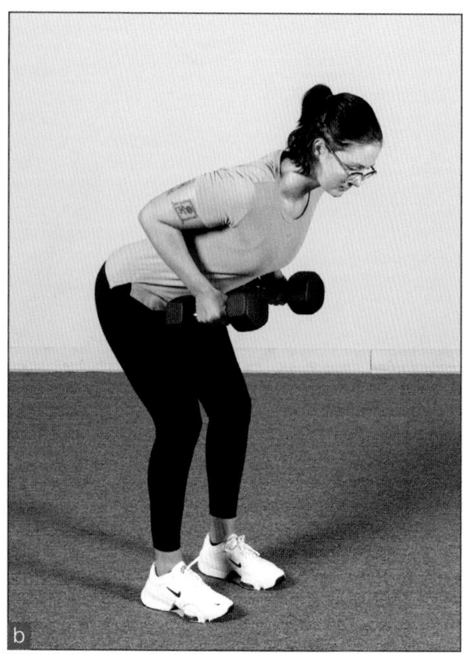
b

1. Stand with your feet hip-width apart, holding a dumbbell in each hand at your side, palms facing each other in neutral position.
2. Hinge at your hips, sliding your dumbbells down your thighs, bending only as far as you can while keeping your spine long. This is your starting position (*a*).
3. Keeping your core engaged and posture strong, pull the dumbbells toward your body. Drive your elbows back toward your hips, squeezing your shoulder blades together and your shoulders away from your ears (*b*).
4. Straightening your arms, lower the dumbbells back down with control, returning to the starting position.
5. Complete the desired number of reps.

## Things to Keep in Mind

- If you are feeling the movement in your lower back, check your posture. It is also OK to do a few reps, stand up, reset, and then go back down into your hinged position.

## Variation

- The dumbbell bent-over row can also be done by alternating one arm at a time.

# SUPPORTED SINGLE-ARM ROW

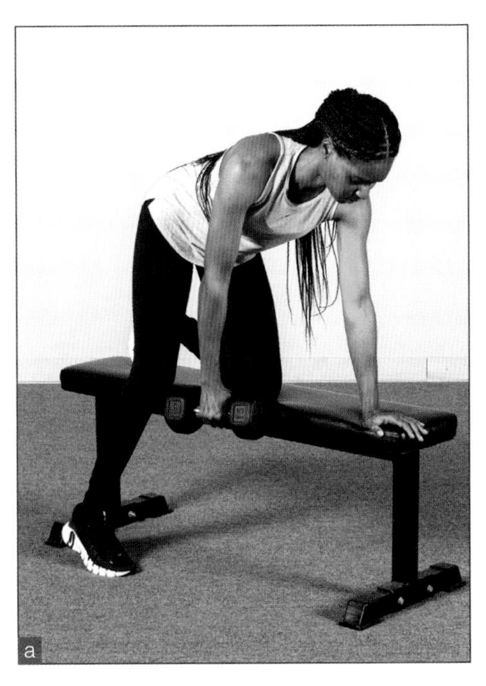
a

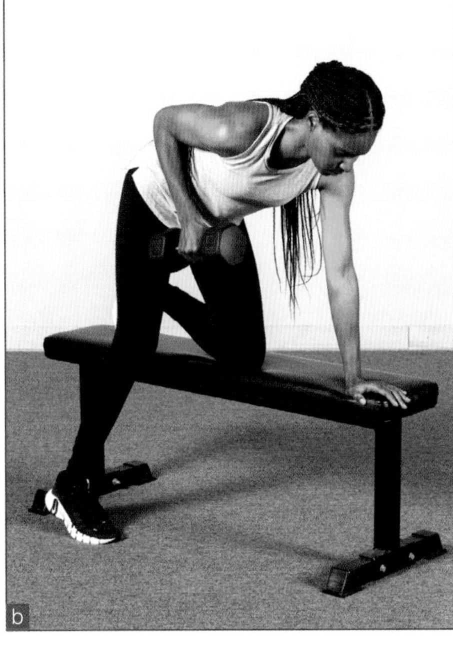
b

1. Place your left hand and the front of your left shin on a sturdy box or bench.
2. Holding a dumbbell with your right hand, extend your arm. Then place your right leg behind you with your knee slightly bent, using the left hand and knee on the box for support (*a*).
3. Hinge at your hips, keeping your spine long. Pull the dumbbell toward your body. Drive your right elbow back toward your hip, squeezing your shoulder blades together (*b*).
4. Slowly lower the dumbbell with control and complete the desired number of reps.
5. Repeat on the other side.

## Things to Keep in Mind

- Keep your abs engaged during the whole exercise, and make sure you are keeping your pelvis neutral. Do not excessively arch your lower back in the supported position.

# SEATED CABLE ROW

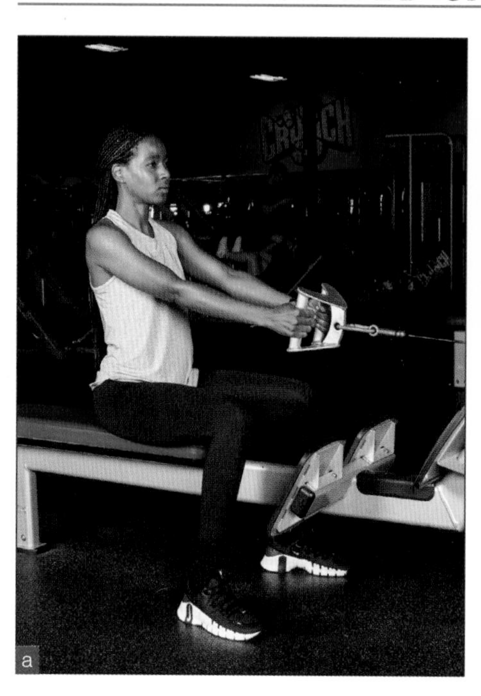

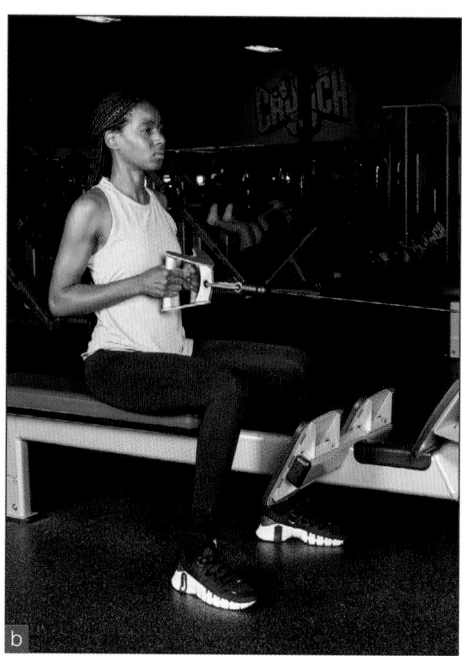

1. Attach a double handle to a cable machine so that you can use it with both hands.
2. Sitting on a box or bench facing the machine, adjust the machine to a middle position so that the handle is in line with your chest
3. Begin with both arms extended, holding a handle in each hand (*a*).
4. Pull the handles toward your chest, driving your elbows back squeezing your shoulder blades together (*b*).
5. Hold for 1 to 2 seconds, then straighten your arms to return to the starting position.
6. Complete the desired number of reps.

## Things to Keep in Mind

- As you bring the handle to your chest, make sure your core is engaged and your shoulders are down. They shouldn't be creeping up toward your ears as though you were shrugging.

## Variations

- The seated cable row can be done with a supinated or neutral grip.
- You can do this exercise in half-kneeling position or tall kneeling position. In half-kneeling position, you can do a single-arm variation, where you move the arm on the same side of the knee that is down. For a tall kneeling position, both knees are down and your hips are extended, like you are "standing on your knees."

# REVERSE FLY

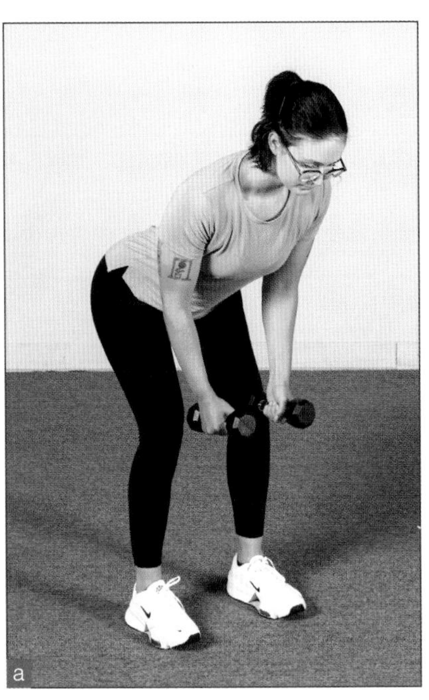


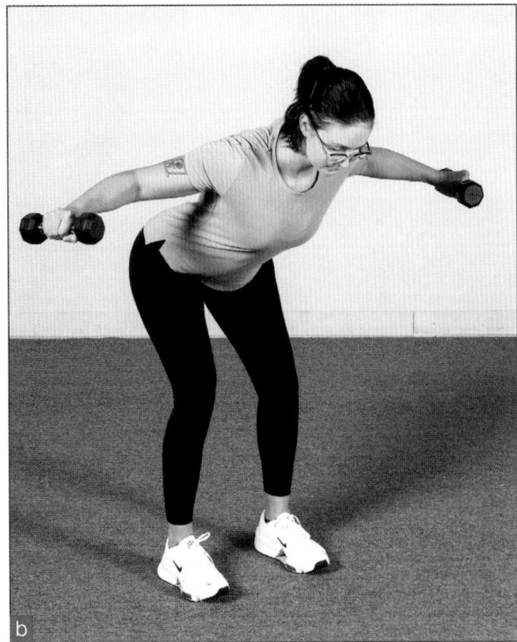


1. Stand with your feet hip-width apart, holding a dumbbell in each hand in front of your thighs, palms facing in.
2. Hinge at your hips, sliding your dumbbells down your thighs, moving only as far as you can while keeping your spine long (*a*).
3. Keeping your core engaged and posture strong, raise your dumbbells out to the sides, away from each other, squeezing your shoulder blades together. Keep your arms as straight as is comfortable; bending your elbows slightly is acceptable (*b*).
4. Lower the dumbbells with control and return to the starting position.
5. Stay in the hinged position and drive elbows back again for the desired number of reps.

## Things to Keep in Mind

- If you are feeling the movement in your lower back, check your posture. It is also OK to do a few reps, stand up, reset, and then go back down into your hinged position.
- Make sure you are moving your arms from in front of you to behind you, instead of at your sides.

## Variations

- The reverse fly can also be done by alternating one arm at a time.
- This exercise can also be done supported like the supported single-arm row on page 119.

# DUMBBELL DYNAMIC HIGH PULL

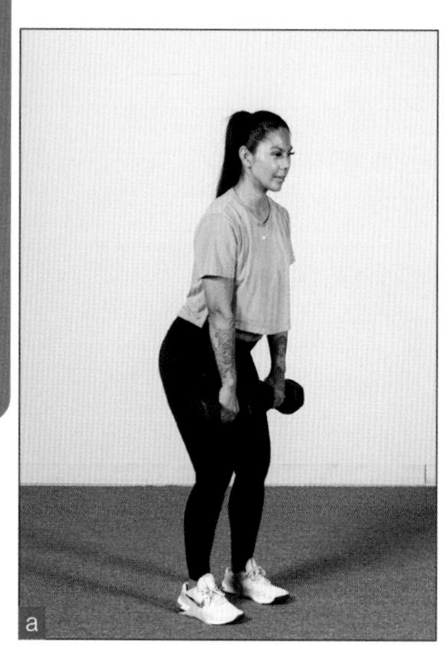
a

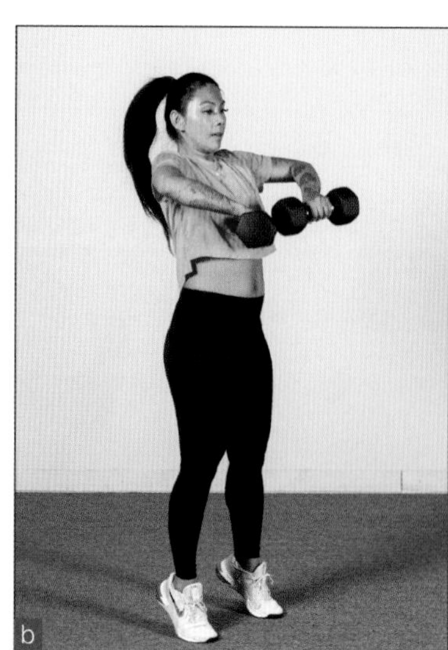
b

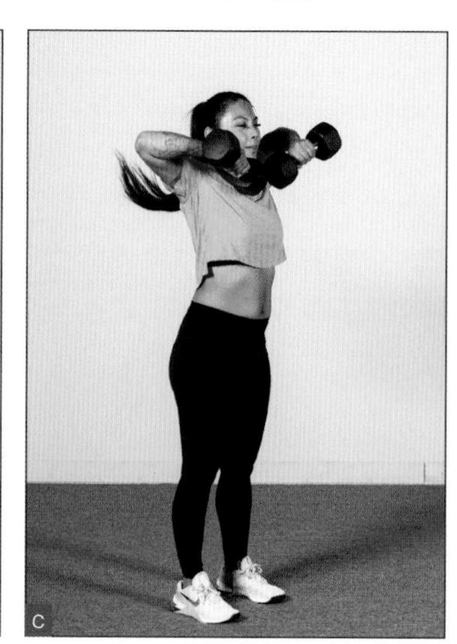
c

1. Stand with your feet hip-width apart, holding a dumbbell in each hand in front of your thighs. Use a pronated (overhand) grip and keep your shoulders back.
2. Bend your knees slightly, and hinge only a few inches, moving your hips back and sliding your dumbbells down your thighs (*a*).
3. With momentum and power, straighten your knees and push your hips forward so that you are standing tall, while simultaneously lifting your heels off the ground, keeping your elbows high, and bringing your dumbbells straight up toward your chin at the range of motion that feels good for you (*b*).
4. Squeeze your shoulder blades together for a second, keeping your core tight (*c*).
5. Lower your dumbbells down to the starting position with control, and complete the desired number of reps.

## Things to Keep in Mind

- You can start with a lighter weight to practice the motion, but the movement should be done with a little momentum, so a heavier weight is usually needed.

# DUMBBELL CLEAN

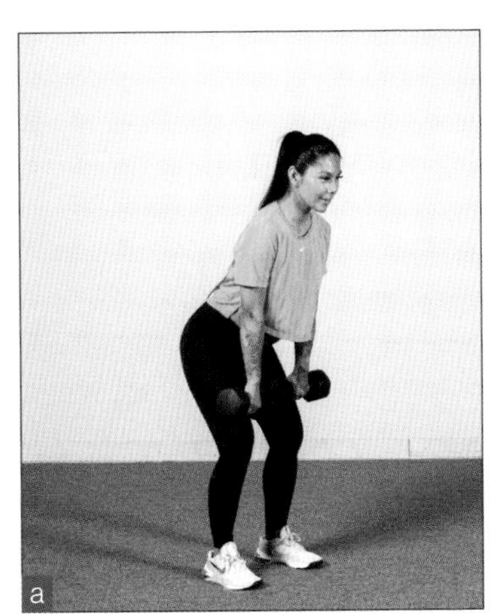


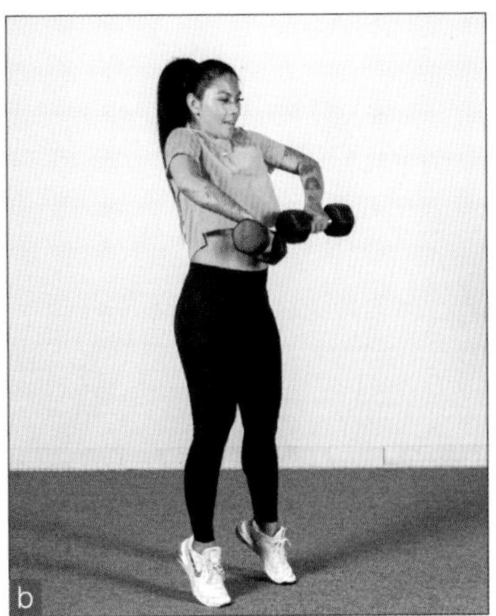


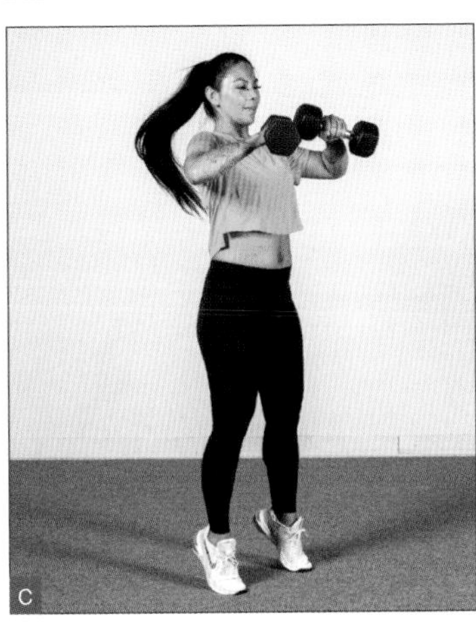


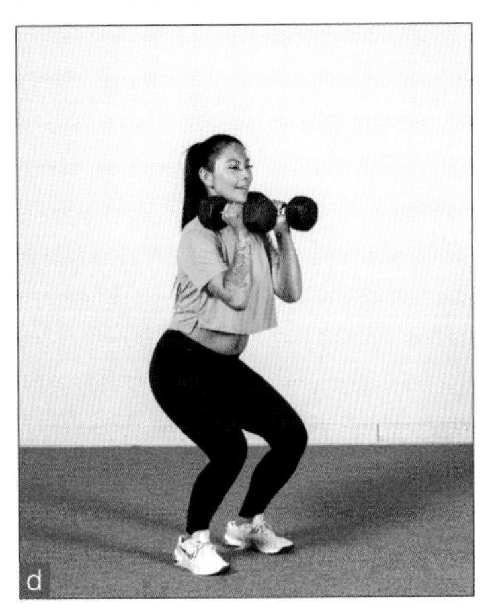


1. Stand with your feet hip-width apart and your shoulders back, holding a dumbbell in each hand with a pronated (overhand) grip in front of your thighs.
2. Bend your knees slightly, and hinge only a few inches, moving your hips back and sliding your dumbbells down your thighs (*a*).
3. With momentum and power, straighten your knees and push your hips forward so that you are standing tall, while simultaneously lifting your heels off the ground, keeping your elbows high, and bringing your dumbbells straight up toward your chin (*b*).
4. Quickly bring your elbows to your side so that your dumbbells rotate (*c*) and end up at your shoulders in a rack position, then bring your heels back down to the ground, keeping your knees soft (*d*).
5. Lower your dumbbells down to the starting position with control, and complete the desired number of reps.

## Things to Keep in Mind

- You can start with a lighter weight to practice the motion, but the movement should be done with a little momentum, so a heavier weight is usually needed.

# DUMBBELL BICEPS CURL

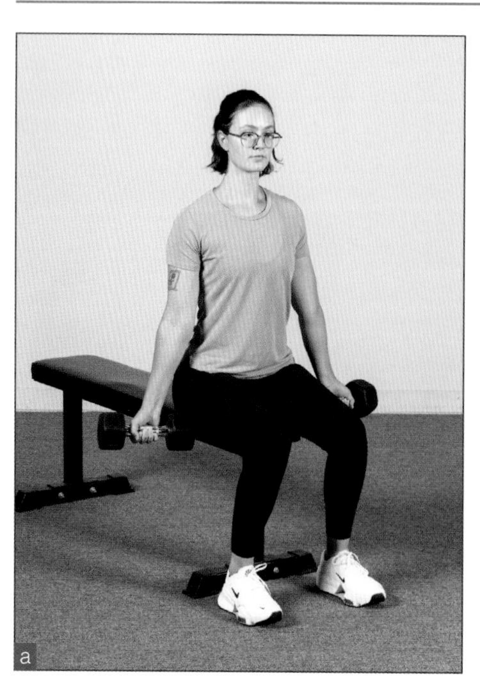
a

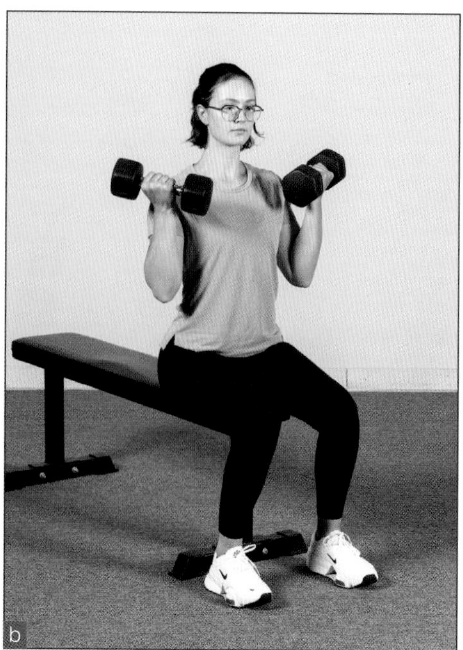
b

1. Sit at the end of a bench or stand. Hold a dumbbell in each hand with your palms facing away from you and your elbows hugged to your rib cage (*a*).
2. Keeping your upper arms motionless, slowly bring the dumbbells up toward your shoulders, moving only from the elbows (*b*).
3. Slowly lower the dumbbells back to the starting position, and complete the desired number of reps.

## Things to Keep in Mind

- Do not swing the dumbbells up to your shoulders.
- Keep your elbows in front of your body, glued to your rib cage. The tendency is to let them creep behind you when the movement gets challenging.

## Variation

- The dumbbell biceps curl can also be done by alternating one arm at a time.

# DUMBBELL HAMMER CURL

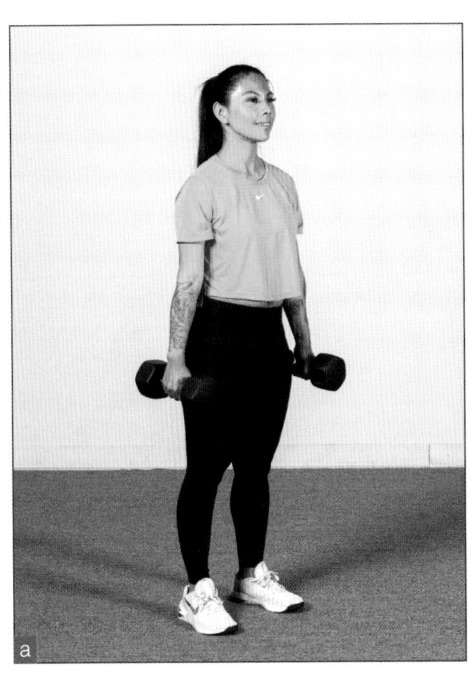
a

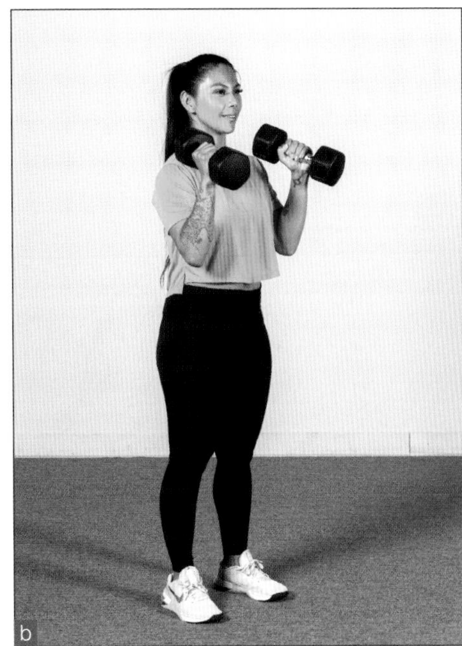
b

1. Sit at the end of a bench or stand. Hold a dumbbell in each hand with your palms facing each other and your elbows hugged to your rib cage (*a*).
2. Keeping your upper arms motionless, slowly bring the dumbbells up toward your shoulders, moving only from the elbow (*b*).
3. Slowly lower the dumbbells back to the starting position, and complete the desired number of reps.

## Things to Keep in Mind

- Do not swing the dumbbells up to your shoulders.
- Keep your elbows in front of your body, glued to your rib cage. The tendency is to let them creep behind you when the movement gets challenging.

## Variation

- The dumbbell hammer curl can also be done by alternating one arm at a time.

## VARIATION OF GRIPS FOR CHIN-UP, PULL-UP, AND PULL-DOWN

For the next three exercises, the unassisted chin-up, superband assisted chin-up, and seated pull-down, you can vary the grips to work different muscles. These will be indicated in each workout in part III, and it is ideal that you stick with the grip that is given, if you are able to do so with the equipment you have. You follow all the same steps; the only difference is you change your grip in step 1 for the unassisted chin-up or step 3 for the assisted chin-up. For the seated pull-down, you may need to adjust the attachment in step 1 that will allow you to have a neutral grip, if it is available to you.

The chin-up with the supinated grip is usually the easiest along with the neutral grip for most people to start with versus the pronated or overhand grip. In a supinated or neutral grip, the biceps are involved a little more than in the pronated grip. In the programs, they can be interchanged if necessary, but try to stick with the programs in order to progress your movements.

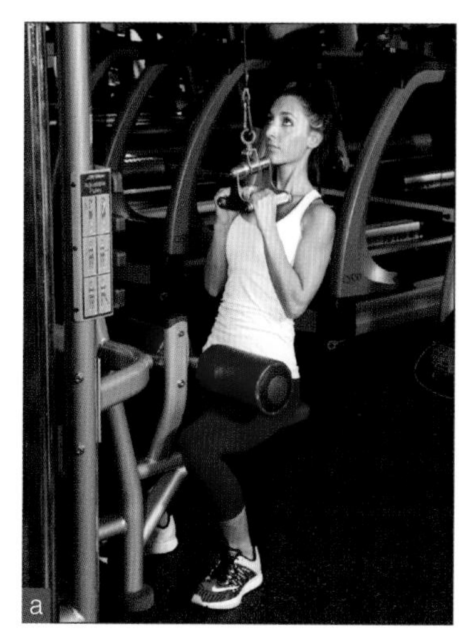

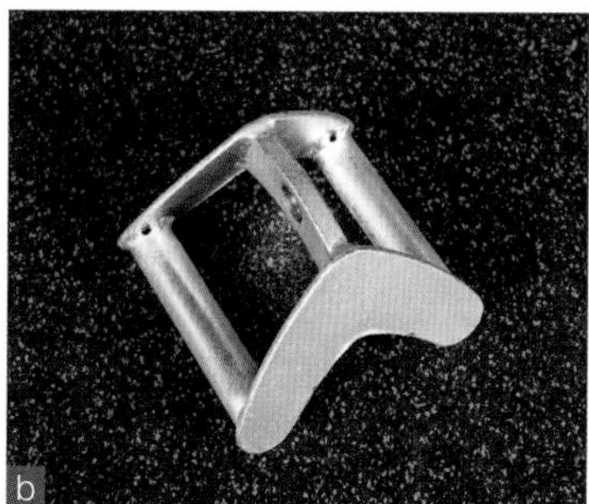

Neutral grip pull-down (*a*) and neutral grip handle (*b*).

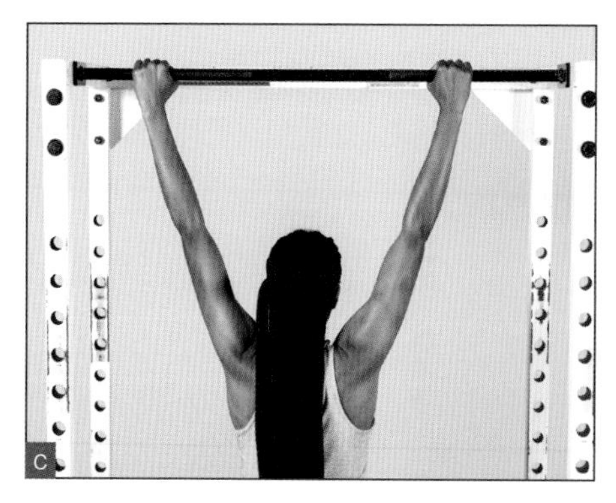

Pronated/overhand grip pull-up (*c*); this is what a typical pull-up looks like.

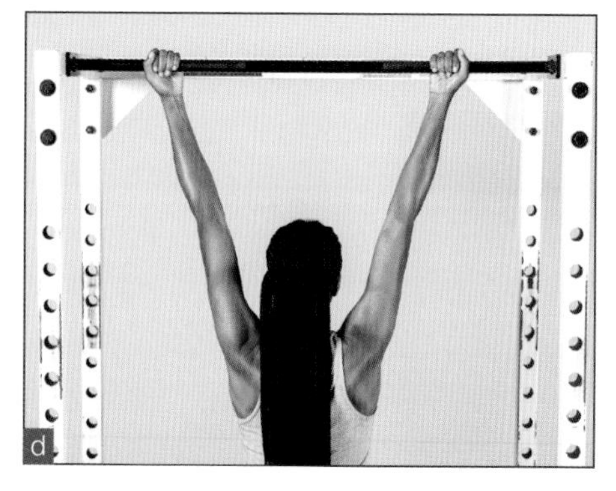

Supinated or chin-up grip (*d*).

# UNASSISTED CHIN-UP

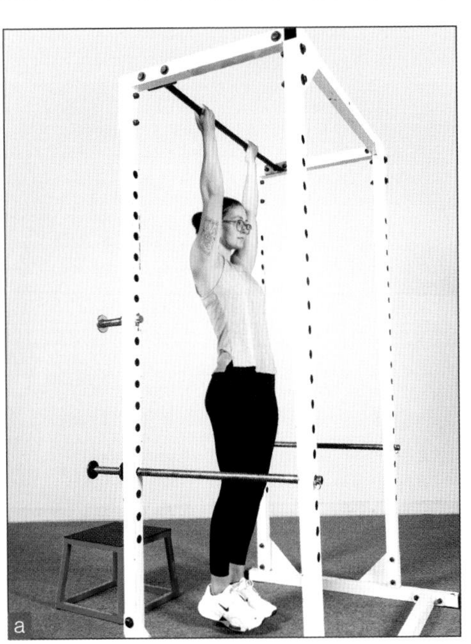

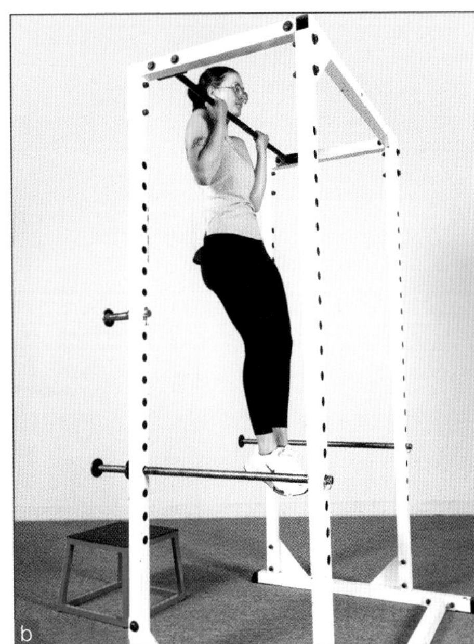

1. Start by standing on a sturdy and safe surface, like a box or bench, facing a pull-up bar.
2. Extend your arms so that you can reach the bar with your hands about shoulder-width apart and a supinated (underhand) grip, so that your palms are facing you.
3. Slowly step off the box or bench, letting yourself hang from the bar fully extended. This is your starting position (*a*).
4. Pull yourself up and over the bar, driving your elbows back, squeezing your shoulder blades together down your back (*b*).
5. Slowly lower yourself back to the starting position, and complete the desired number of reps.

## Things to Keep in Mind

- Don't do half reps by lowering yourself only halfway; extend your arms completely by lowering yourself all the way down.
- Make sure you are on a sturdy surface to safely reach the bar. If you feel comfortable jumping up to the bar, make sure you can do so safely.
- Do not allow your shoulders to creep up by your ears; if this happens, modify by using a light superband as shown in the superband assisted chin-up (the next exercise).

## Variations

- The unassisted chin-up can be done with a pronated or neutral grip.
- An isometric hold can be done by jumping up and holding onto the bar. Even if you hold on for less than 5 seconds, this is a great way to progress to the chin-up.

# SUPERBAND ASSISTED CHIN-UP

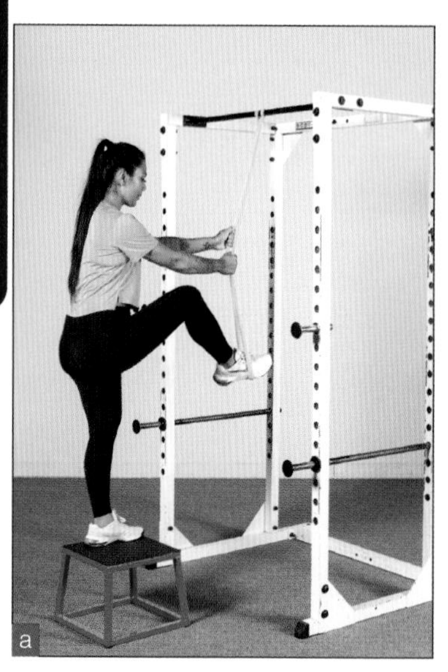
a

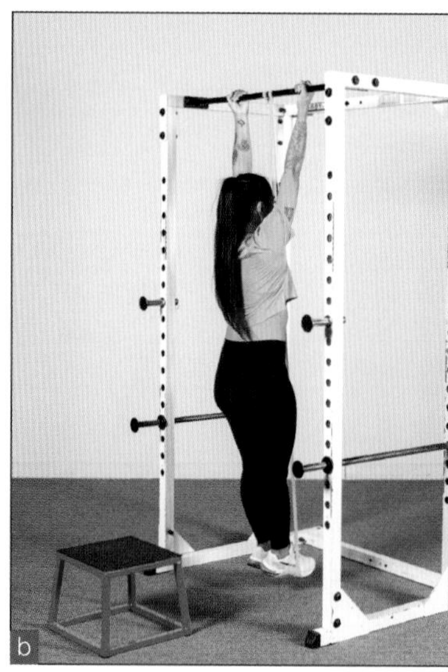
b

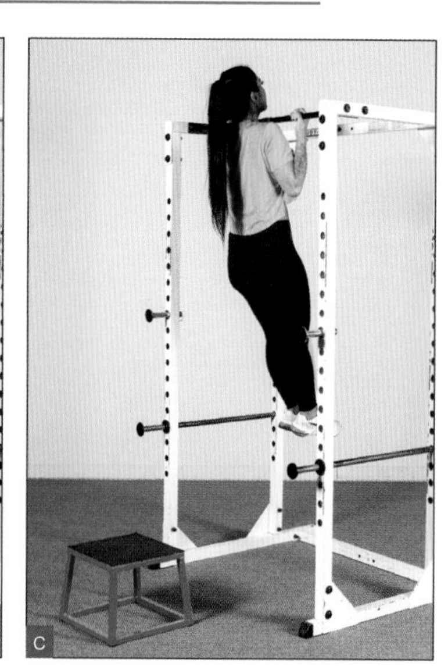
c

1. Start by standing on a sturdy and safe surface, like a box or bench, facing a pull-up bar, with a superband hooked around the pull-up bar. The thicker the superband is, the more assistance you will have. Of course the opposite is true too: the thinner the superband, the more challenging this exercise will be.
2. Place one foot inside the superband loop (*a*).
3. Once you are hooked into the superband, grip the bar with both hands, using a supinated (underhand) grip. Hang from the bar, letting your legs extend, and cross the free leg over the leg that is hooked into the superband (*b*).
4. Repeat steps 4 and 5 of unassisted chin-up (*c*).
5. Complete the desired number of reps, then step the free leg back on the box and use one hand to help unhook you from the superband.

## Things to Keep in Mind

- Don't do half reps by lowering yourself only halfway; extend your arms completely by lowering yourself all the way down.
- Make sure you are on a sturdy and solid surface to safely reach the bar. You may need someone to help you get in and out of the superband.
- Do not allow your shoulders to creep up by your ears, if this happens, modify by using a thicker superband.

## Variations

- The superband assisted chin-up can be done with a pronated or neutral grip.
- An isometric hold can be done by jumping up and holding. Even if you hold for less than 5 seconds, this is a great way to progress to the chin-up.

# SEATED PULL-DOWN

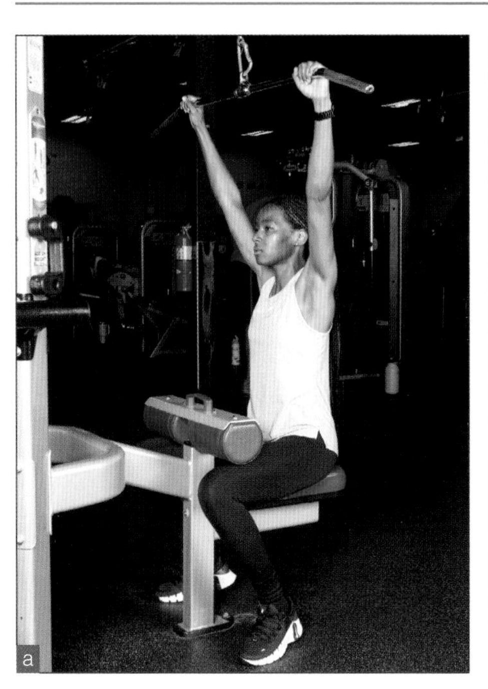
a

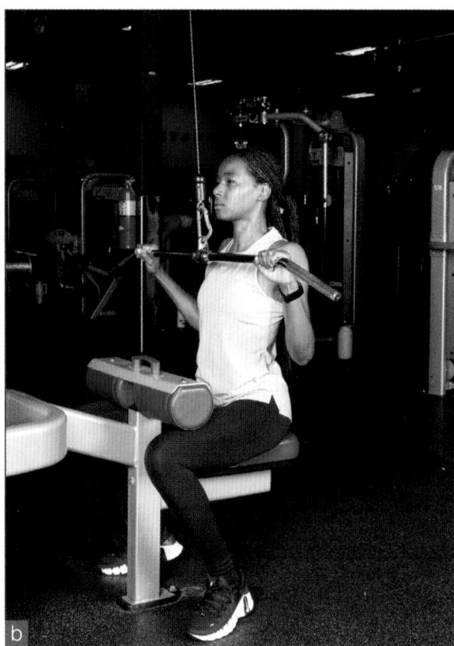
b

1. Find a cable machine that has a seat or space that you can move a box or bench to, and attach a bar that is long enough for you to grip at about shoulder height when seated.
2. Adjust the cable machine so that the handle is high enough for you to extend your arms overhead while in a seated position using a pronated (overhand) grip (*a*).
3. Pull the bar down toward your chest, driving your elbows down and squeezing your shoulder blades together (*b*).
4. Hold for 1 to 2 seconds, then straighten your arms to return to the starting position.
5. Complete the desired number of reps.

## Things to Keep in Mind

- As you bring the bar to your chest, make sure your core is engaged so you do not excessively extend or arch your lower back.

## Variations

- The seated pull-down can be done with a supinated or neutral grip.
- You can do this exercise in half-kneeling position or tall kneeling position, rather than sitting on a bench or box.

# SINGLE-ARM PULL-DOWN

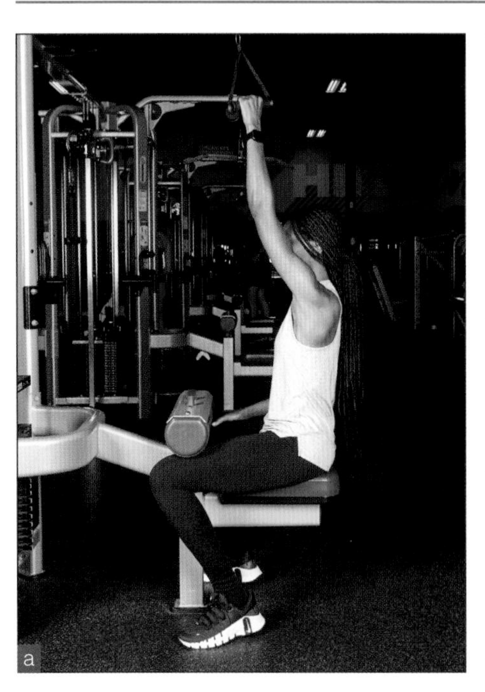

a

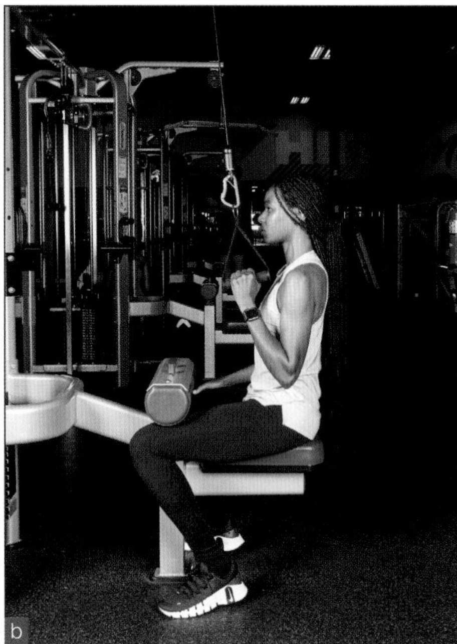

b

1. Find a cable machine that has a seat or space that you can move a box or bench to, and attach a handle that is long enough for you to grip at about shoulder height while seated.
2. Adjust the cable machine so that the handle is high enough for you to extend your arm overhead while in a seated position (*a*).
3. With a pronated (overhand) grip, pull the handle down toward your armpit, driving your elbow down your back and squeezing your shoulder blades together (*b*).
4. Hold for 1 to 2 seconds, then straighten your arm to return to the starting position.
5. Complete the desired number of reps, then repeat on the other side.

## Things to Keep in Mind

- As you bring the bar to your chest, make sure your core is engaged so you do not excessively extend or arch your lower back.

## Variation

- You can do the single-arm pull-down in half-kneeling position or tall kneeling position. In the half-kneeling position, remember that if your left knee is on the floor, then you should hold the cable in your left hand, and vice versa.

# SCAPULAR PULL-UP

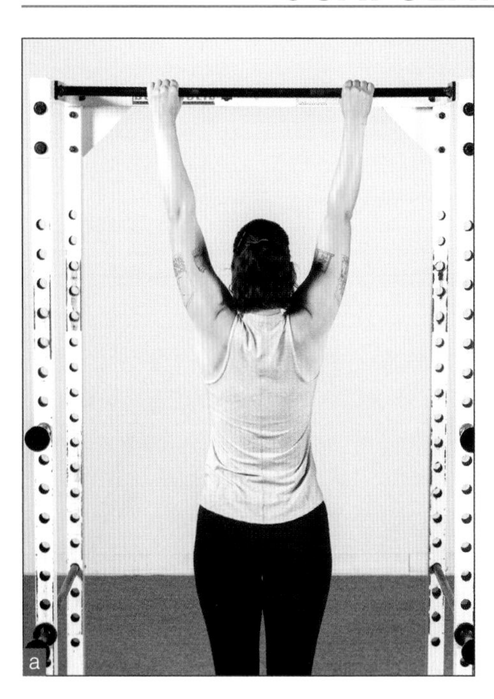


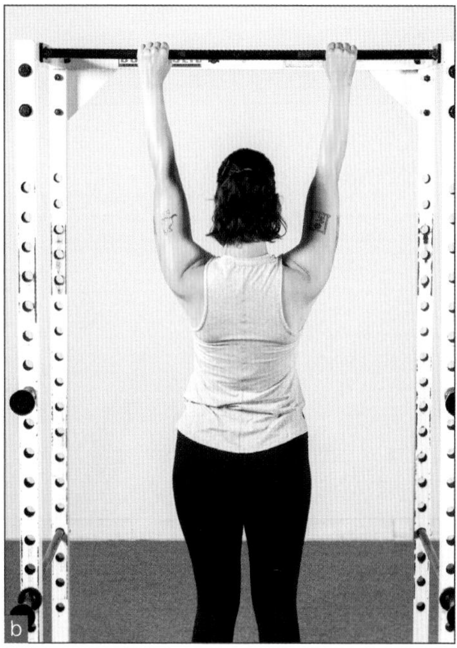


1. Start by standing on a sturdy and safe surface, like a box or bench, facing a pull-up bar.
2. Extend your arms so that you can reach the bar with your hands about shoulder-width apart and a pronated (overhand) grip, so that your palms are facing away from you.
3. Slowly step off the box or bench, letting yourself hang from the bar fully extended. This is your starting position (*a*).
4. While hanging and keeping your arms straight, pull your shoulders down as you lift yourself closer to the bar, squeezing your shoulder blades together, holding for 1 to 2 seconds or the desired amount of time (*b*).
5. Complete the desired number of reps.

## Things to Keep in Mind

- If you are still working on improving your grip, it's OK to come down from the bar and do one or two reps, then repeat.

# MODIFIED PULL-UP

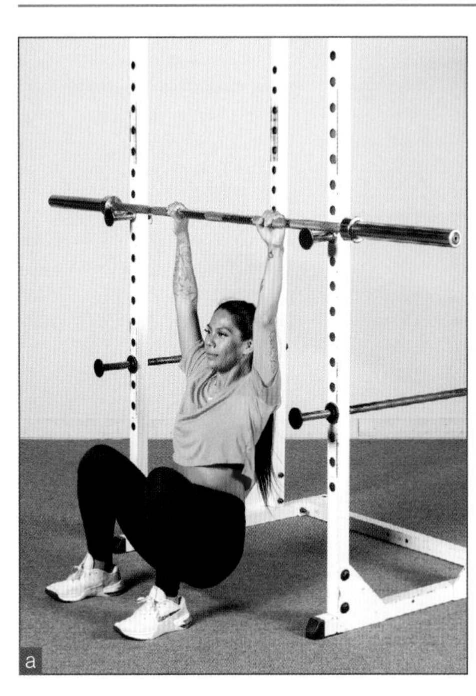
a

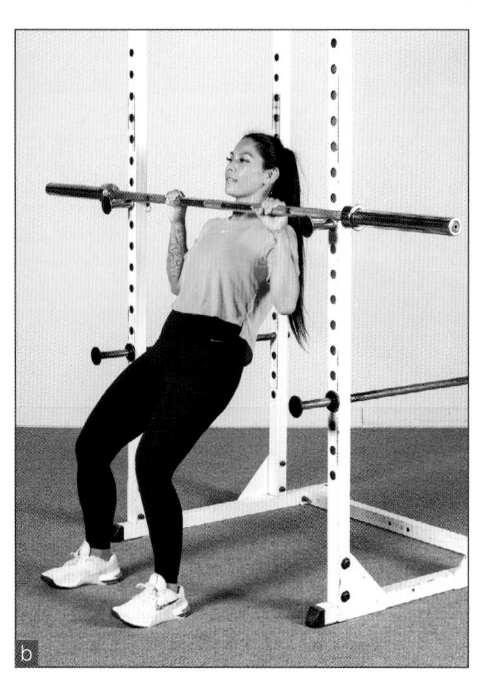
b

1. Set up a barbell in a high position so that if you were seated underneath it, your arms can fully extend overhead.
2. Sit directly under the bar on a sturdy bench or box, if necessary.
3. Extend your arms overhead and grip the bar about shoulder-width apart with a pronated (overhand) grip (*a*).
4. Without using your legs too much, pull yourself up to bring your chest to the bar, driving your elbows down and squeezing your shoulder blades together (*b*).
5. Hold for 1 to 2 seconds and then lower yourself back down with control; complete the desired number of reps.

## Things to Keep in Mind

- Make sure the bar you have set up is sturdy enough so that it can't move while you are gripping it from underneath.
- Make sure your arms are extended overhead so that you are doing a vertical pull, pulling yourself vertically toward the bar.

## Variation

- The modified pull-up can be done with a supinated grip.

# 9

# TOTAL BODY AND ROTATIONAL EXERCISES

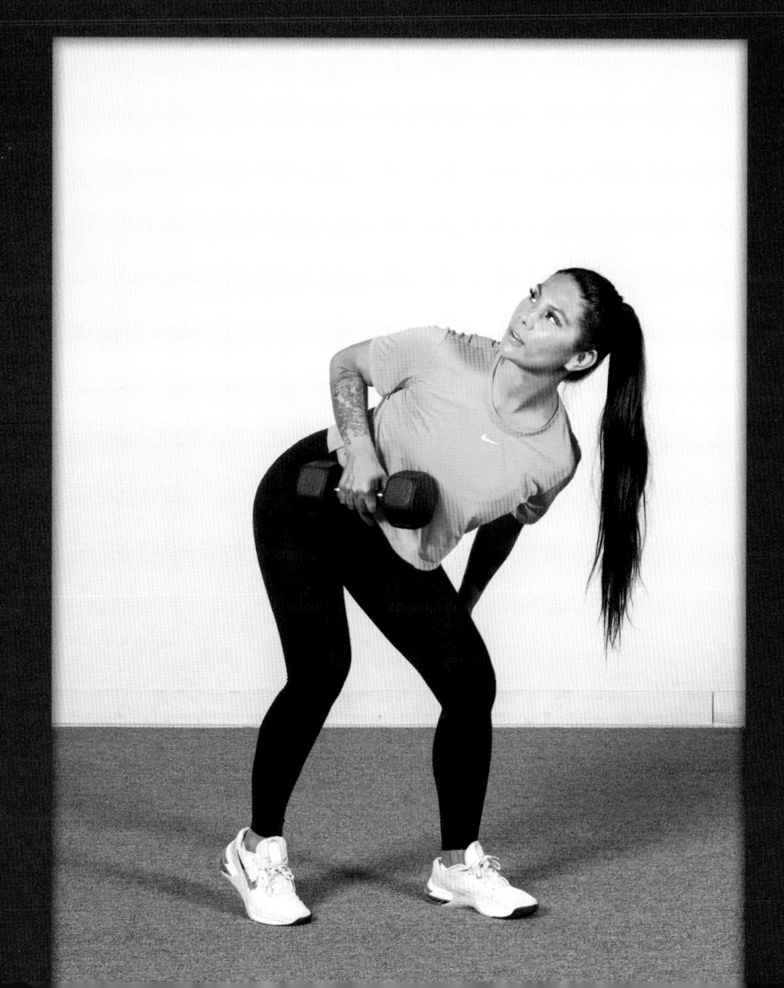

This chapter features exercises that have some of the same movement patterns as those in the preceding chapters, but work the total body. And, while chapter 5 includes antirotational core movements, this chapter has a few rotational exercises that are more controlled and some that are dynamic, where you use a little more momentum.

These moves are vital to a regular strength-training routine because they improve your proprioception, or body movement awareness, and boost your overall functionality. Most of these can get your heart rate up, but you likely won't be lifting really heavy weight with them. These exercises can be warm-ups, done at the end of a circuit or superset, or used to finish the workout.

# STANDING LOW TO HIGH LIFT

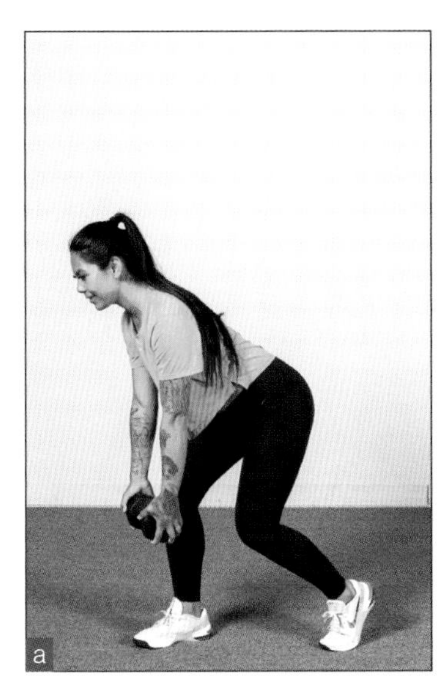
a

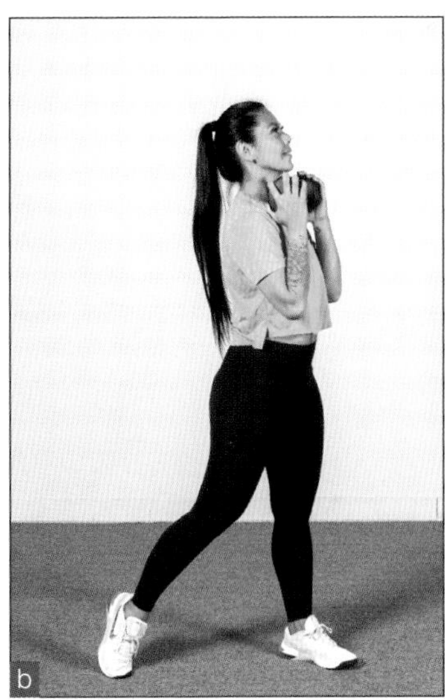
b

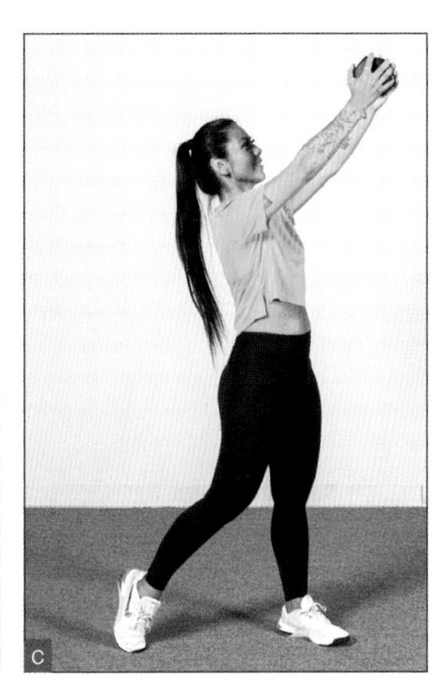
c

1. Stand with your feet about hip-width apart, using both hands to hold one dumbbell in front of your chest.
2. Straighten your arms as you lower the dumbbell to your right knee, lifting your left heel and pivoting it outward slightly, making sure you keep your spine long (*a*).
3. Bend the elbows and bring the dumbbell back to the starting position at your chest as you return to standing and start to pivot in the other direction (*b*).
4. Straighten your arms again as you press and lift the dumbbell overhead to your left, lifting your right heel and pivoting it outward (*c*).
5. Bend the elbows as you lower the dumbbell back to the starting position at your chest. This is one repetition.
6. Complete the desired number of reps, then repeat on the other side.

## Things to Keep in Mind

- Try this exercise as a body-weight movement first, then add the dumbbell.
- Allow your body to naturally rotate in whichever direction you are facing by pivoting your feet.

# STANDING DYNAMIC LOW TO HIGH LIFT

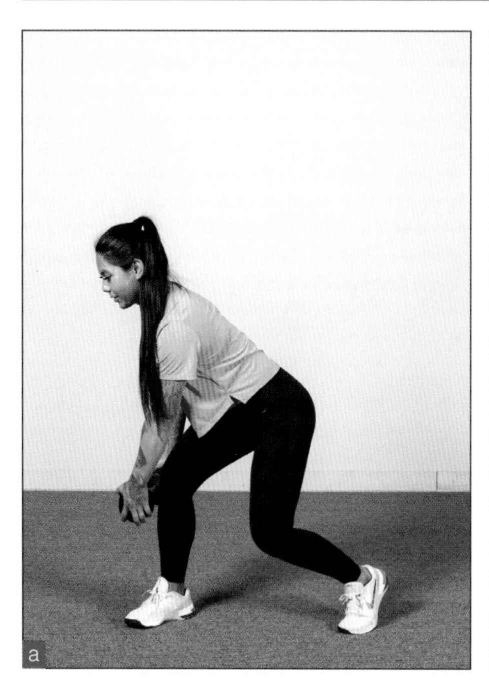
a

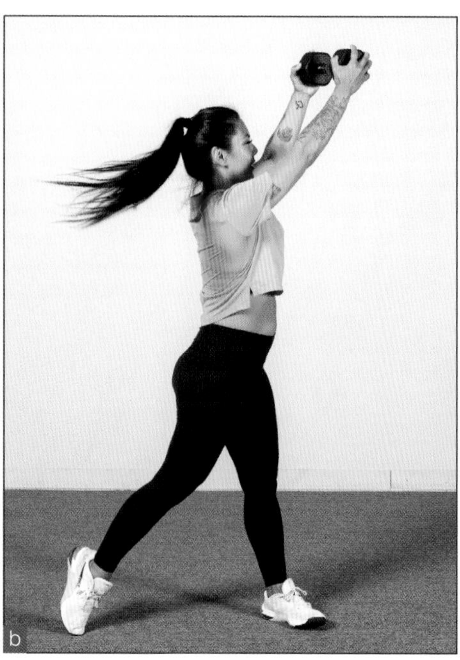
b

1. Complete steps 1 and 2 of standing low to high lift (*a*).
2. Dynamically lift your dumbbell up to your right side, keeping your elbows slightly bent, rotating your upper body slightly and pivoting your left heel outward (*b*).
3. Lower and return to the starting position with control.
4. Complete the desired number of reps, then repeat on the other side.

## Things to Keep in Mind

- Do not rush this movement—it's not about getting each repetition done quickly.
- Keep your abs engaged as you move through the lift, allowing yourself a powerful exhale as you dynamically move through the lifting motion.

# HALF-KNEELING LOW TO HIGH LIFT

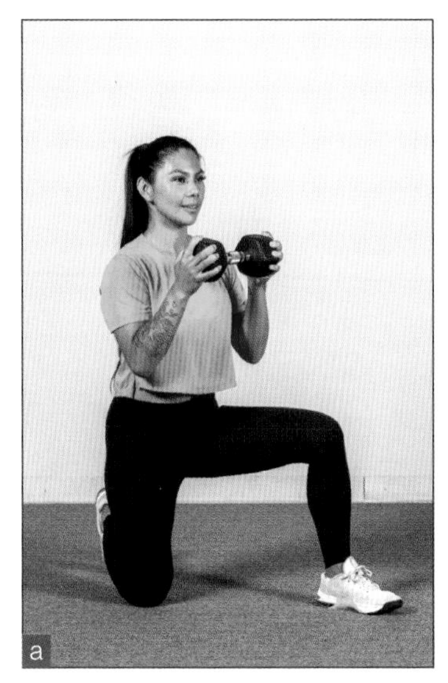
a

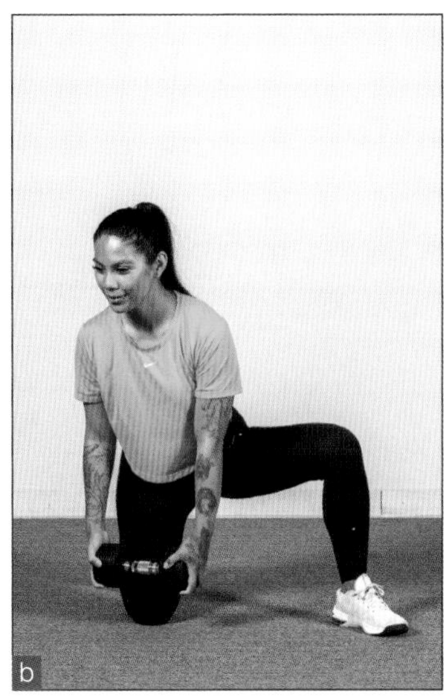
b

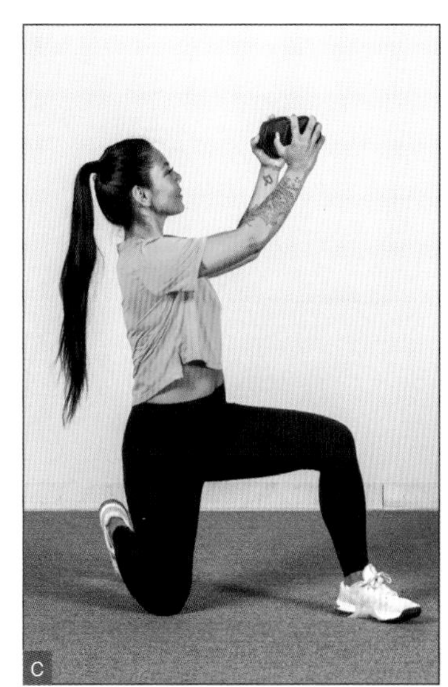
c

1. Start with your right knee on the ground and your left knee bent at a 90-degree angle so you are in a half-kneeling position, making sure your stance isn't too narrow. Your right toes should be curled under, so that your foot is flexed. If your flexibility does not allow this, the top of your foot can be flat on the ground.
2. Use both hands to hold one dumbbell in front of your chest, with elbows bent (*a*).
3. Hinge at your hips, lowering your hips toward your heel, and lowering the dumbbell toward your right knee as your arms straighten, making sure you keep your spine long (*b*).
4. Extend your hips back to the starting position as you bend the elbows and bring the dumbbell back to your chest.
5. Rotate the upper part of your spine as you straighten your arms, lifting the dumbbell up to your left side (*c*).
6. Bend the elbows as you lower the dumbbell back to the starting position at your chest, and complete the desired number of reps.
7. Repeat on the other side.

## Things to Keep in Mind

- Try the exercise as a body-weight movement first, then you can add the dumbbell.

# HALF-KNEELING DYNAMIC LOW TO HIGH LIFT

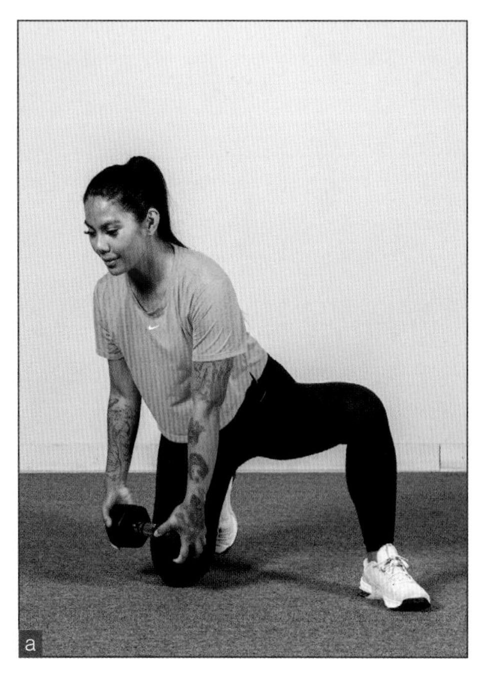
a

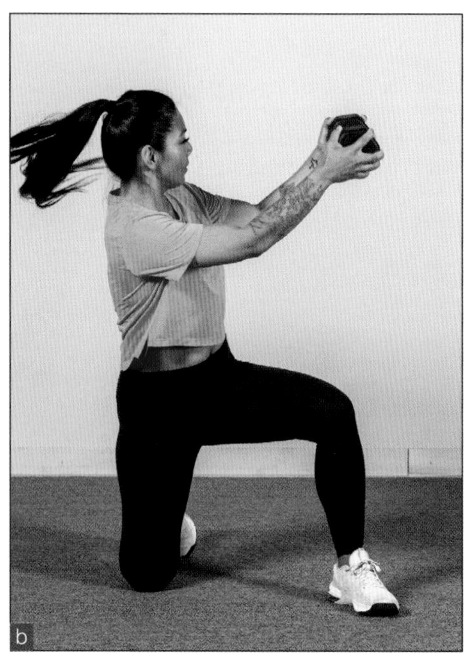
b

1. Start with steps 1 through 4 of half-kneeling low to high lift (*a*).
2. Dynamically drive your hips forward to the starting position, as you swing the dumbbell over your left shoulder with control, keeping your elbows slightly bent (*b*).
3. Lower the dumbbell back to the starting position with control, and complete the desired number of reps.
4. Repeat on the other side.

## Things to Keep in Mind

- Do not rush this movement. It's not about getting each repetition done quickly.
- Keep your abs engaged as you move through the lift, allowing a powerful exhale as you dynamically move through the lifting motion.

# REVERSE LUNGE TO DYNAMIC LIFT

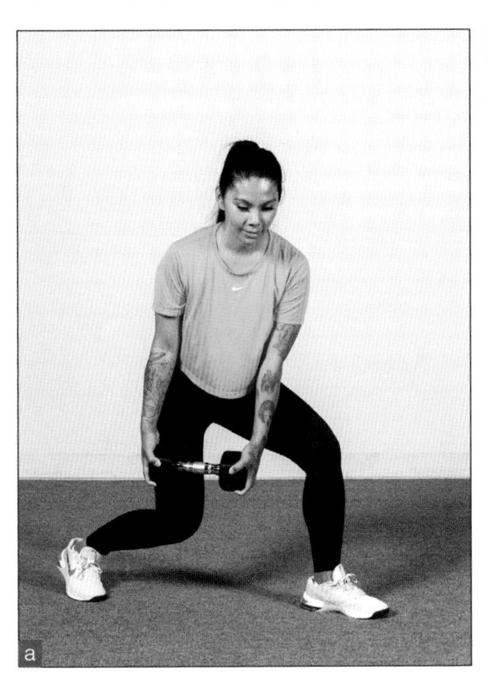
a

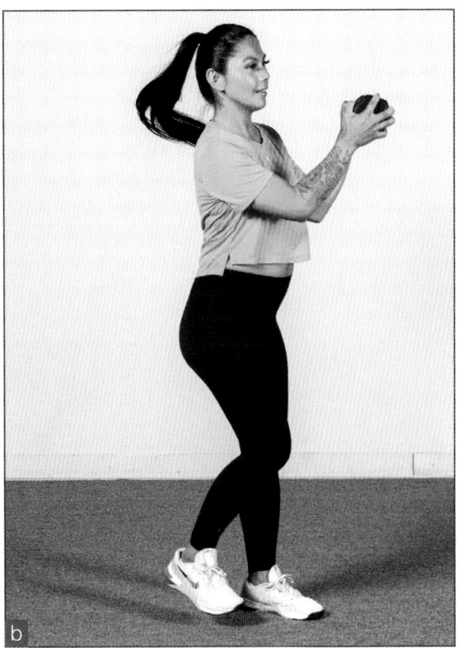
b

1. Stand with your feet hip-width apart, and use both hands to hold one dumbbell in front of your chest.
2. Step your right foot back into a reverse lunge, bending your knees, as you straighten your arms and lower your dumbbell toward your right knee, slightly rotating the upper part of your back (*a*).
3. Drive through your left heel to return to your standing position, while simultaneously lifting the dumbbell up toward your left shoulder, bending both elbows (*b*).
4. Complete the desired number of reps.
5. Repeat on the other side.

## Things to Keep in Mind

- Do not rush this movement. It's not about getting each repetition done quickly. Make sure to pause briefly after each lift, then step back slowly into the next lunge.
- Keep your abs engaged as you move through the chop, allowing a powerful exhale as you dynamically move through the lifting motion.

# ROTATIONAL OVERHEAD PRESS

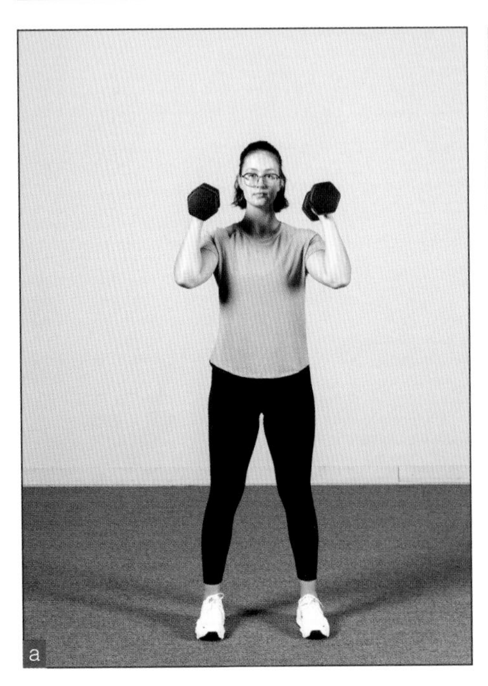
a

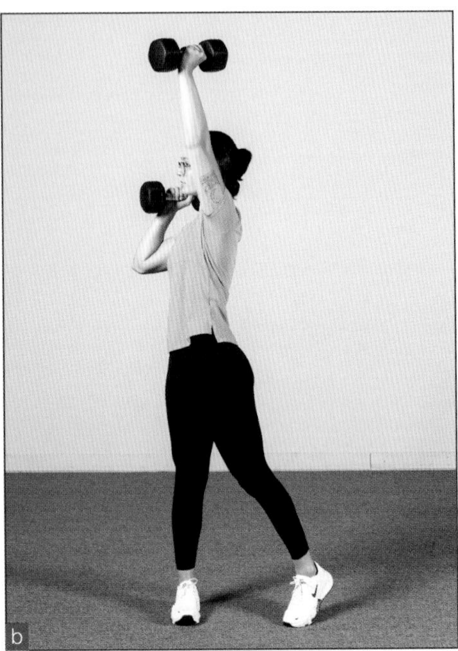
b

1. Start with your feet hip-width apart and hold a dumbbell in each hand.
2. Bring your dumbbells in line with your shoulders with your elbows bent and your palms facing each other (*a*).
3. Lift your left heel and turn your body to your right, as you press your left dumbbell straight overhead, extending your arm completely (*b*).
4. Slowly lower with control as you rotate back to your starting position.
5. Lift your right heel and turn your body to your left, as you press your right dumbbell straight overhead, extending your arm completely.
6. Slowly lower with control as you rotate back to your starting position. This is one repetition. Complete the desired number of reps.

## Things to Keep in Mind

- Make sure you press the dumbbell straight up above your body, rather than away from your body.
- Allow your body to naturally rotate in whichever direction you are facing by pivoting your opposite foot in that direction.

# ALTERNATING STEP BACK TO CURL AND PRESS

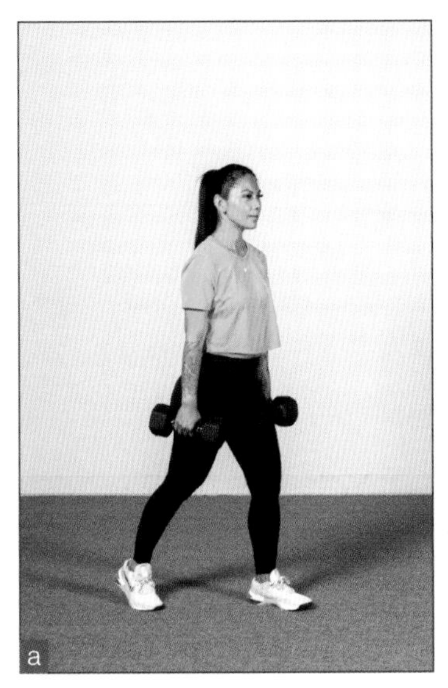

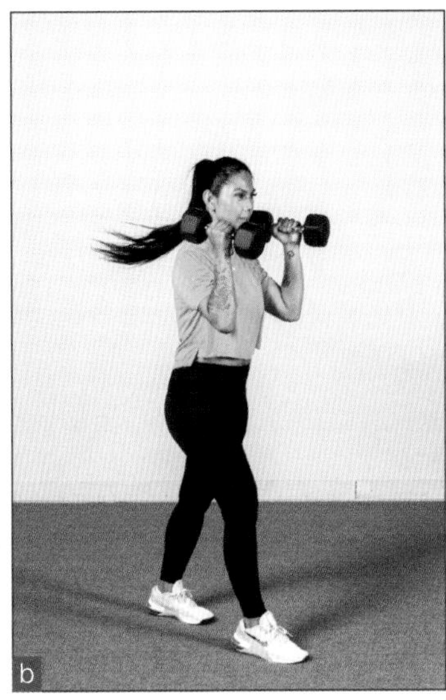

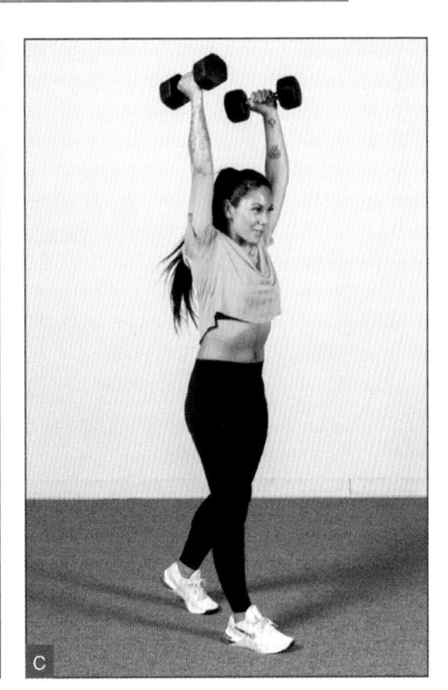


1. Start in a staggered stance with your right foot slightly behind the left, holding one dumbbell in each hand at your side (*a*).
2. Step your right foot forward as if you were walking, while simultaneously curling your dumbbells to your shoulders in a neutral grip (*b*).
3. Keeping that stance, press both dumbbells overhead, straightening your arms so that your biceps are in line with your ears (*c*).
4. Lower your dumbbells to your sides with control as you bring both feet under your hips, and then repeat on the other side. This is one repetition.
5. Alternate for the desired number of reps.

## Things to Keep in Mind

- Do not rush this movement. After you perform the press, slowly reset back at the middle and start the next rep.
- Exhale powerfully on the press and use a little momentum.

# ALTERNATING PLANK ROW

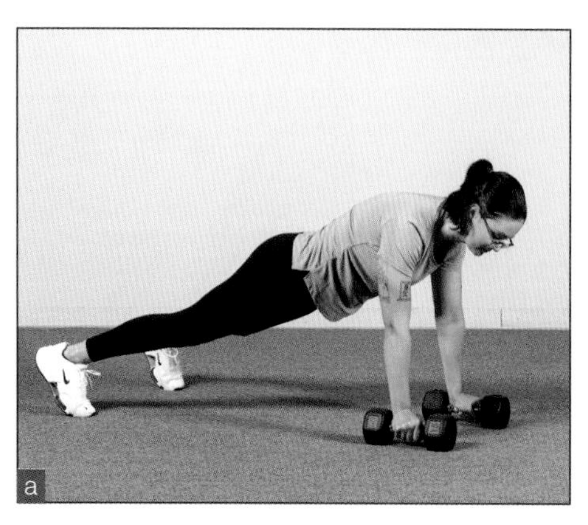
a

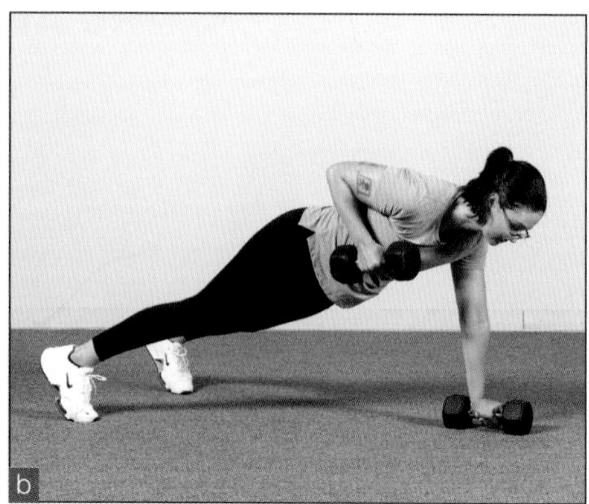
b

1. Start in a high plank position, holding a dumbbell in each hand, palms facing in. You can fully extend your legs or place the knees on the floor. In either position, the feet or knees should be about hip width apart (*a*).
2. Lift one dumbbell off the ground, driving your elbow back toward your hips and up toward the sky in a horizontal pull, keeping your hips level (*b*).
3. Lower with control back to the starting position and repeat on the other side. This is one repetition.
4. Complete the desired number of reps.

## Things to Keep in Mind

- Keeping your feet or knees wider apart in this movement increases stability.
- Pretend you are balancing something on the small of your back and you can't let it spill; this may help you to keep your hips level throughout the movement.

# SQUAT TO OVERHEAD PRESS

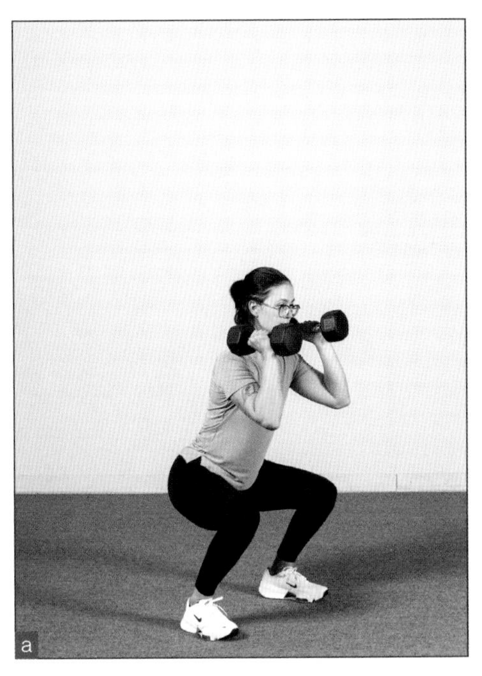
a

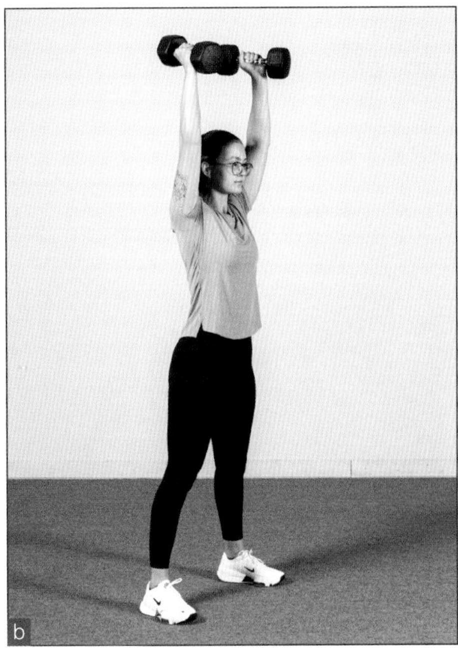
b

1. Stand with your feet hip-width apart, holding a dumbbell in each hand in the rack position at your shoulders, and elbows hugged in toward your rib cage.
2. Bend your knees, lowering into a squat, keeping your posture tall and core engaged (*a*).
3. Stand back up, and with the momentum of the squat, press both dumbbells overhead, straightening your arms so that your biceps meet your ears (*b*).
4. Lower your dumbbells back to the starting position with control and complete the desired number of reps.

## Things to Keep in Mind

- Use the momentum from your squat to press your dumbbells overhead, but do not blend each rep into the next.
- Take your time to reset at the start position before beginning the next rep.

# HINGE TO ROW ROTATION

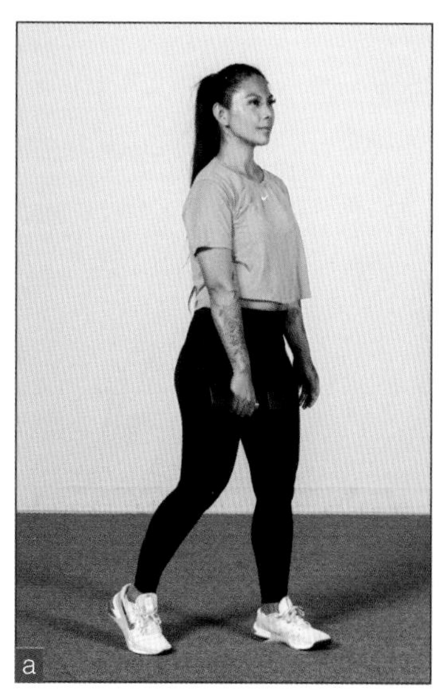
a

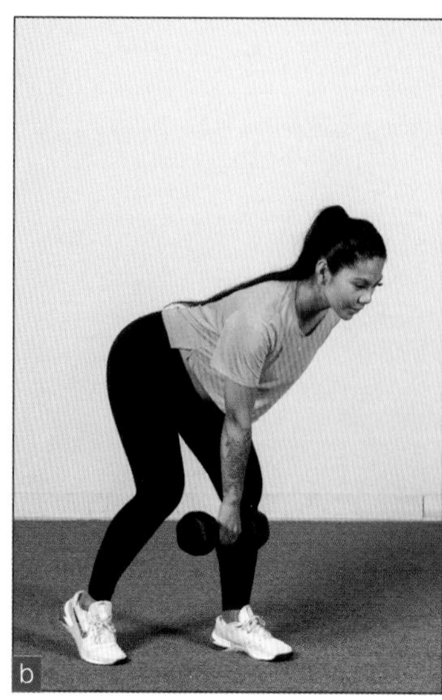
b

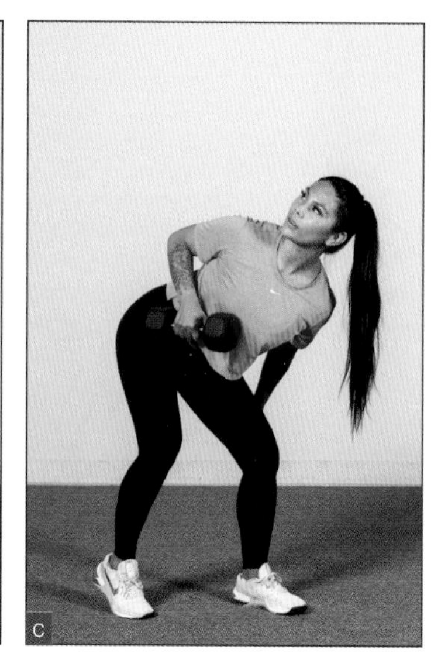
c

1. Stand with your feet hip-width apart holding a dumbbell in your right hand, your arm extended and the dumbbell held in front of your right thigh.
2. Slide your right foot back about 6 inches (15 cm), with your heel lifted so that you are in a staggered or "kickstand" position (*a*).
3. Hinge slowly at your hips as you lower your dumbbell toward the floor, rotating slightly to your left, bringing the dumbbell toward your left shin, making sure your core is engaged (*b*).
4. Rotate your head to the right, and drive the dumbbell back to your right hip, keeping your elbow close to your side (*c*).
5. Slowly stand back up with control, and complete the desired number of reps.
6. Repeat on the other side.

## Things to Keep in Mind

- Keep your core engaged for the whole time, and allow yourself to rotate slightly at the bottom of the movement, turning your upper body in the appropriate direction.

# CABLE HIGH TO LOW CHOP

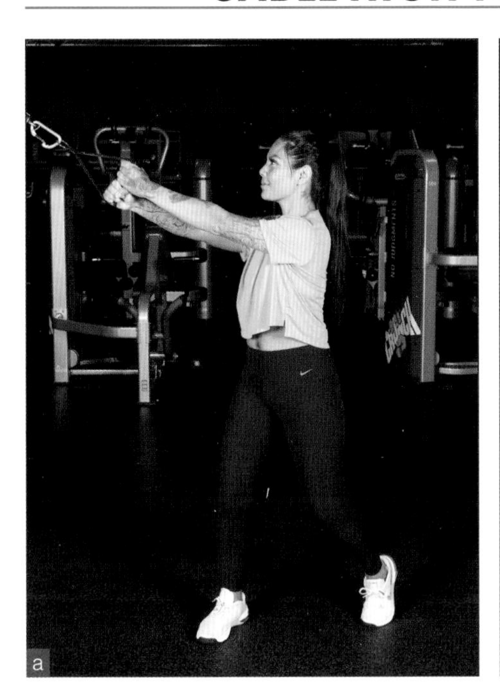
a

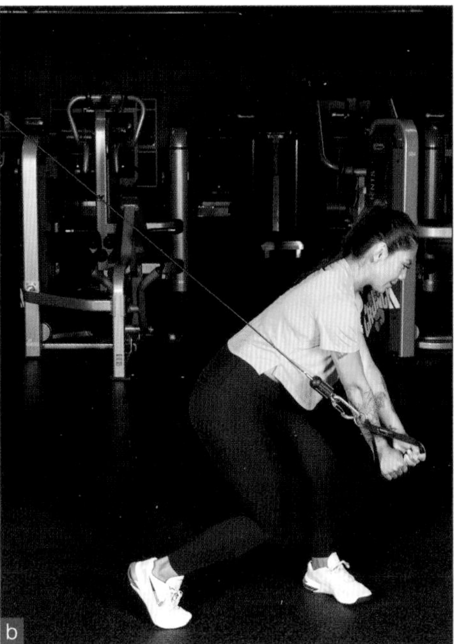
b

1. Stand with your cable or superband anchored at a high angle and orient yourself so that you are perpendicular to the anchor and your right foot is closest to the anchor. Grab the handle or superband with both hands and walk away slightly so that there is tension in the cable and your arms are extended at an angle up and to your right, keeping your left heel lifted and pivoted toward your right (*a*).
2. Dynamically lower the cable or superband down toward your left knee, keeping your arms straight and pivoting your right foot, lifting that heel and rotating your upper body (*b*).
3. Bring the cable or superband back up to the starting position with control, and complete the desired number of reps.
4. Repeat on the other side.

## Things to Keep in Mind

- Exhale as you bring the cable or superband down.
- Do not rush the movement; reset after each rep.

# STAGGERED CABLE TWIST

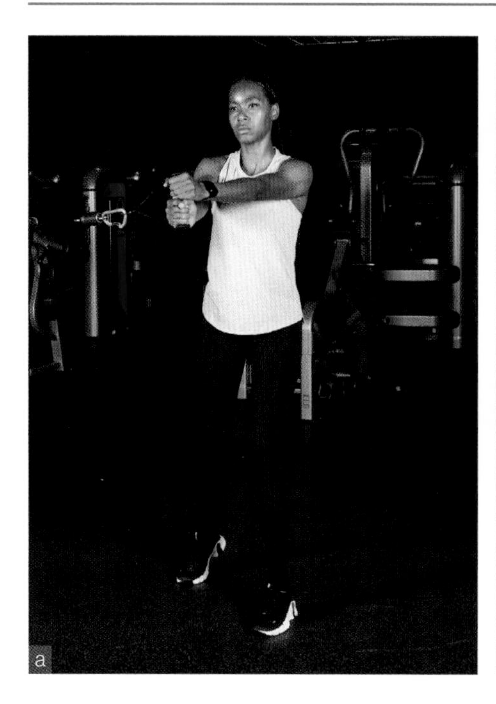
a

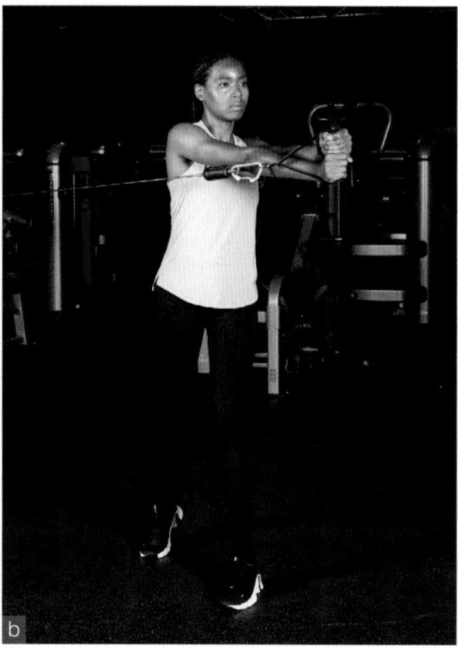
b

1. Stand with a cable or superband anchored in line with your chest and orient yourself so that you are perpendicular to the anchor, with your right foot closest to the anchor.
2. Grab the handle or superband in both hands and walk away slightly so that there is tension and your arms are straight in front of your chest.
3. Stand in a staggered position so that your right foot is back; this is your starting position (*a*).
4. Keep your feet planted as you rotate your upper body to your left, keeping your arms straight, and letting a slight rotation happen in your hips, but not so much that you become unstable (*b*).
5. Complete the desired number of reps, and repeat on the other side.

## Things to Keep in Mind

- Control the cable instead of chopping it.
- Allow the twist to come from your upper body.
- Do not lean in the direction that you are twisting.

# SQUAT TO ROW

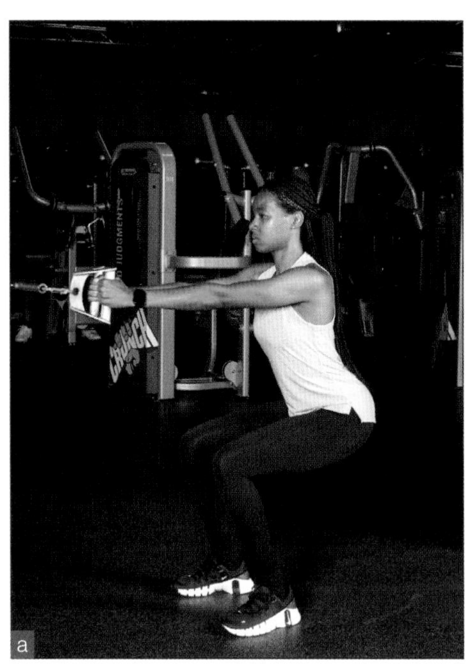
a

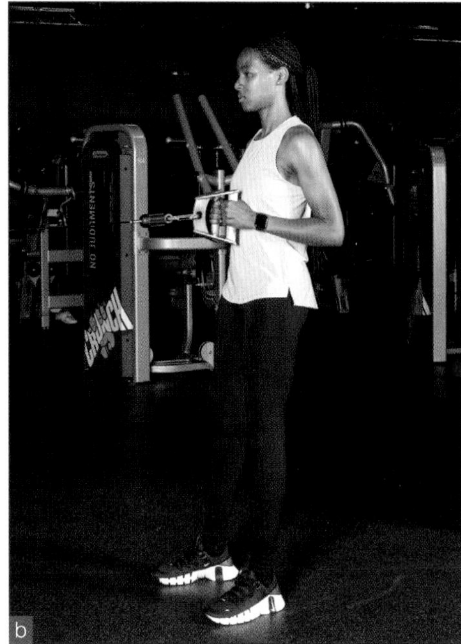
b

1. Stand with a cable or superband anchored in line with your chest and orient yourself so that you are facing the anchor.
2. Grab the handle or superband with both hands and walk yourself far enough back so that there is a little tension when your arms are straight.
3. Bend your knees, lowering down into the squat, keeping your arms straight out in front of you (*a*).
4. As you stand up, pull the handles toward you, driving your elbows back and squeezing your shoulder blades together (*b*).
5. Complete the desired number of reps.

## Things to Keep in Mind

- Try not to lean back as you do your row at the top. Use your abs to keep your posture tall.

# PRONE BACK EXTENSION

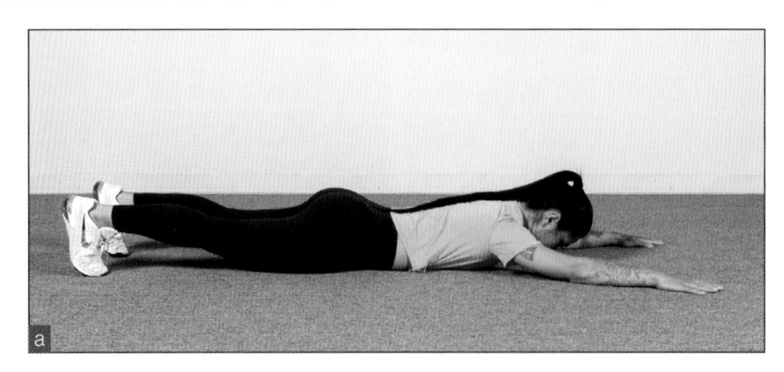

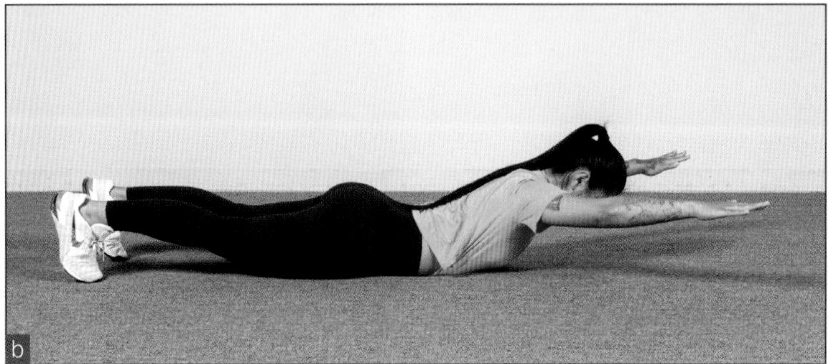

1. In a prone position (lying on your front), extend both arms over your head and flat on the ground. Flex your feet so that your toes are pushing into the ground (*a*).
2. Lift your chest and hands off the ground so that the upper part of your body is lifted, while keeping your feet on the ground. Your glutes should be engaged (*b*).
3. Hold for 1 to 3 seconds, then lower back down with control.
4. Complete the desired number of reps.

## Things to Keep in Mind

- Keep your glutes and core engaged to make sure you are not hyperextending your lower back.
- The focus should be on lifting your chest off the ground and making the movement come from your upper and middle back.

## Variation

### Prone W Back Extension

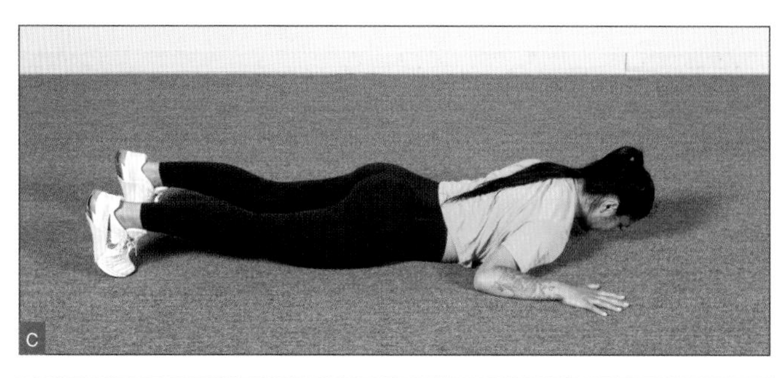


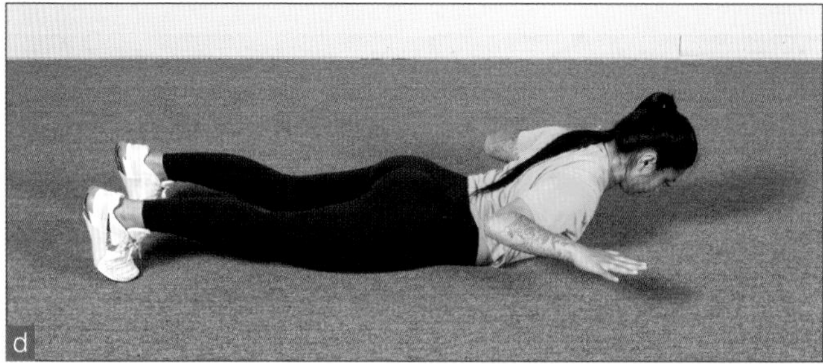


1. In a prone position (lying on your front), bend your elbows, keeping your hands flat on the ground, creating a W with your arms. Flex your feet so that your toes are pushing into the ground (*c*).
2. Repeat steps 2 through 4 of prone back extension (*d*).

## Things to Keep in Mind

- Keep your glutes and core engaged to make sure you are not hyperextending your lower back.
- The focus should be on lifting your chest off the ground and making the movement come from your upper and middle back.

# CABLE PLANK PULL

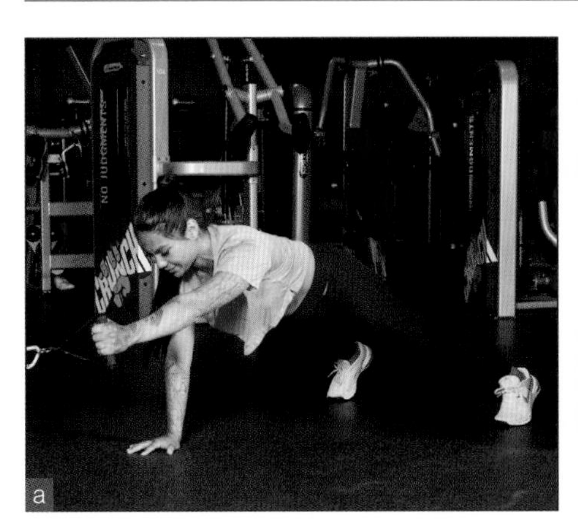

a

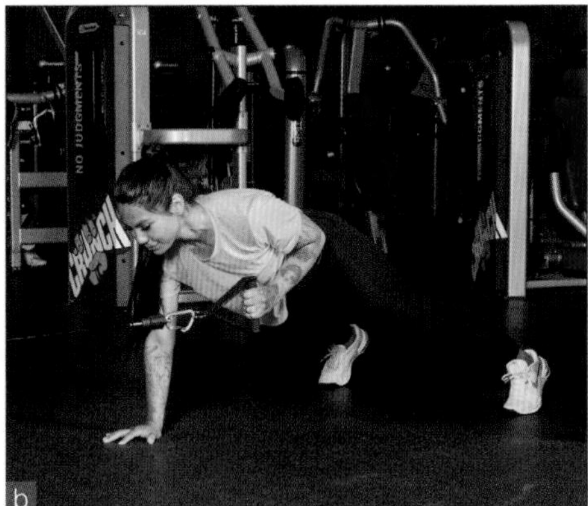

b

1. Set up a cable or band with one handle so that it is anchored in a low position, in line with your shoulders when you are positioned in a high plank.
2. Position yourself back far enough so there is tension in the cable or band when your arm is fully extended and you are in a high plank.
3. Set yourself up in your high plank position, resting on your knees or with the legs fully extended, keeping your knees or feet hip-width apart.
4. Hold the cable or band in one hand, using your other arm to support you in your high plank position. This is your starting position (*a*).
5. Pull the cable toward you with your hand in a neutral position, driving your elbow back toward your hips in a vertical pull, squeezing your shoulder blade back. Keep your hips level (*b*).
6. Fully extend your arm to return to the starting position, and complete the desired number of reps.
7. Repeat on the other side.

## Things to Keep in Mind

- Keeping your feet or knees wider apart in this movement increases stability. Pretend you are balancing something on the small of your back and you can't let it spill; this will help you to keep your hips level.

# PART III

# PROGRAMMING FOR SUCCESS

# 10

# CREATE YOUR OPTIMAL PROGRAM

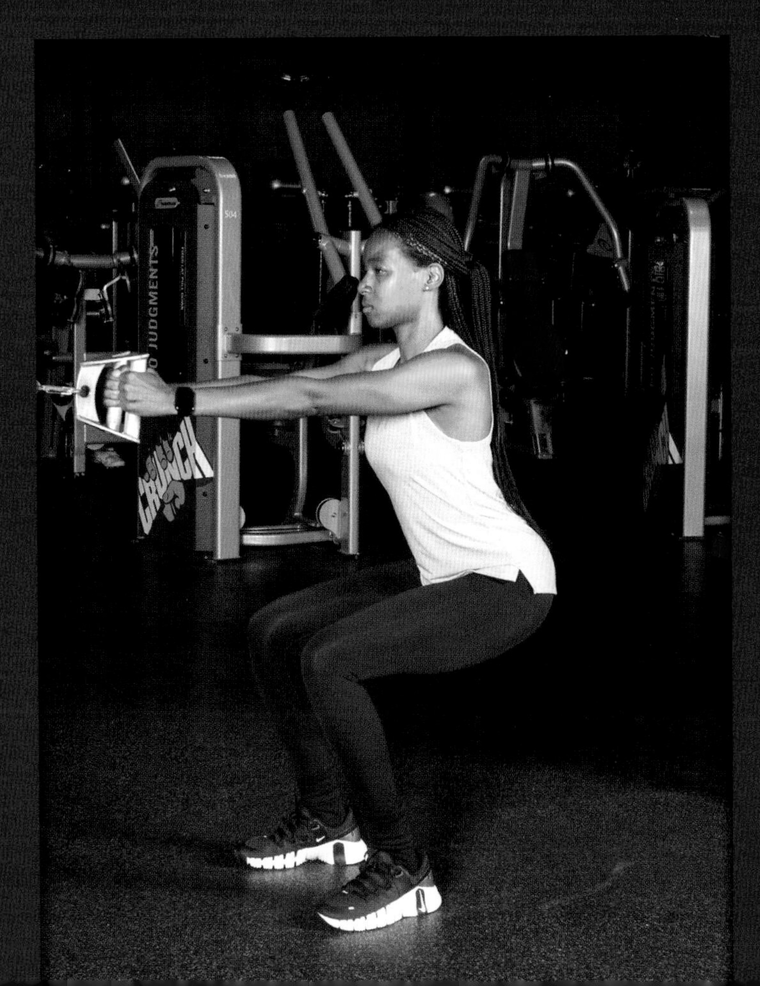

In this book, there are four different programs, each tailored to your goals and the equipment that is available to you. This chapter contains an overview of each program. No matter how familiar or unfamiliar you are with fitness and strength training, there is something for you! Even as a seasoned workout enthusiast and fitness professional, I would find any of these programs beneficial to my own routine, depending on where I am in terms of fitness. You may want to look back at chapter 4, Getting Started, to revisit how to assess your fitness level and how to set SMART goals. If you are still unsure of your SMART goals, this chapter may help you get more dialed in. Let's look at the descriptions to see what fits you best.

## DETERMINING LOAD

It's difficult to know what weight to choose for each exercise if you are just getting started. In these programs, I recommend recording your rate of perceived exertion (RPE) after each exercise until you get a good idea of how the weights feel to you. RPE is based on a 1 to 10 scale, where 1 is the easiest, something you can do practically without a second thought, like an easy stroll down the street; 5 is moderate—your muscles are working hard or your heart rate is above resting, but you are able to do the movement for about 5 more reps or 20 seconds longer; and 10 is the most difficult—you feel completely breathless at the end of the movement, or your muscles are so fatigued that you aren't able to complete the rep.

Each workout includes a recommended number of repetitions for each exercise—for example, 12 to 15 repetitions of an overhead press. When beginning the program and doing that exercise for the first time, pick a weight and aim for the 15 reps. Check in with yourself afterward, and if your RPE feels like a 4 or 5, then the weight may be too easy. The goal is for the weight to feel like a 7 or 8. If your RPE is between 1 and 5, it's OK to do the exercise again with a slightly heavier weight. If the weight is challenging enough for you to feel like you're at an RPE of 7 or 8 at 12 reps, you have picked a good weight! Using the overhead press as an example again, let's say you're able to use 10 pounds (4.5 kg) for three weeks, doing 12 reps each time. By the second week, you feel like you can do 12 reps at an RPE of 5 or 6! This is a good indicator to raise your weight to 12.5 pounds (5.6 kg) for your third week, and so on.

In other training guides, you may see something called a "deloading week." "Deloading" can be described as a period of time when your body gets a little rest because you reduce the loads and/or overall volume of your program, yet you are still lifting on a schedule. This allows your body to recover and make strength gains so that you can be even stronger the following week. I did not schedule these into your programs, though. Realistically, we all know life happens. There may be a week when you are sick, or you're traveling, or you don't have access to a gym that has the equipment you need. Count any of these as your deloading week! Then you can pick up your program where you left off. If you are able to complete all 12 weeks of a program without a break (which I find very rare!) be aware that in the fourth or fifth week, you may need to use lighter loads to allow your body to properly recover for the following week. Again, this is only if you know for sure you can complete all 12 weeks in a row.

## WARM-UPS AND COOL-DOWNS

Warming up and cooling down are important factors in your training routine. The programs in this book include core activations and some body-weight versions of the moves that are intended to function as warm-ups. "Warming up" can mean many things to many people, though. Some people talk about hopping onto a treadmill to warm up for a few minutes. There is nothing wrong with this, especially if you typically take a while to get the juices flowing. Nevertheless, a great way to warm up for a strength workout is to do a dynamic mobility routine that emulates some of the movements in that day's workout. For example, if you are doing a lower-body workout, then you should focus on mobility through your hips and knees. It's beneficial even to do some movements, such as a squat, with just your body weight. You can find some great mobility and warm-up routines in *Smarter Workouts* by Pete McCall (Human Kinetics, 2019).

After your workout, it's important to let your body cool down. Take a few minutes and do some easy static stretching and deep breathing. In static stretching, you hold the stretch for more than 15 seconds. Incorporating deep breathing helps you relax into the stretch. Allowing your body to take that extra time after a workout can help reduce soreness and generally help you relax.

## INCORPORATING OTHER EXERCISE

The programs in this book are focused solely on strength training, with some metabolic training that involves strength exercises. While I strongly advocate for all women to perform strength training at least 2 or 3 times a week, I understand that there are a lot of other modalities of exercise. More important, I am most happy if more of the world is moving! So if you want to incorporate Pilates or a spin or treadmill class, go for it! It's important that you not overdo it, though. Two programs in this book are designed for those who like to take group fitness classes or incorporate a recreational sport. With any of the four programs, you can supplement with Pilates or yoga routines that incorporate mobility and core training, but keep in mind that Pilates and yoga can both be forms of strength training. Listen to your body and adjust your training schedule as needed so that you are not overworking yourself.

If you would like to incorporate more cardio into your routine, there are a few ways you can do that, depending on your goals. Many strength and fitness coaches will argue that one way is better than others, but I disagree. Different methods work for different people. Generally, if you are training for overall strength, I'd recommend tacking on cardiovascular exercise at the end of your workout. Cardio may fatigue you, making it more difficult to do your workout or hit a PR. Additionally, if you want to burn calories, the best time to do your cardio is after strength training because of the increased metabolic rate created by a strength workout. But if you're training for a distance race or just focused on some form of cardio as "your" sport, then it may be better to do your running or cycling before getting into your strength training. Or perhaps you're a busy parent who has to squeeze in a run in the morning and a gym workout in the evening. That's OK too! Because there are so many different variables, there is no absolute right or wrong way to do this.

## CHOOSING A PROGRAM

I've provided you with four different programs that are all 12 weeks long, with 3 to 5 workouts per week. Each program comprises 3 to 5 phases and each is intended to take from 45 minutes to about an hour and 15 minutes. The workouts can be done on consecutive days, or you can do one workout, rest the next day, and then complete the second workout. Don't overthink it; my best advice is to complete them to the best of your scheduling abilities. But make sure you schedule them into your calendar just like any commitment!

Each program has different goals and the gym equipment you have access to should be taken into consideration. These programs are meant to be a guide and can be adjusted accordingly. If you have taken time off because of illness or injury, avoid motivation-sapping comparisons to where you were before. If you do end up having to skip a week or adjust a few days, you can simply pick up where you left off and adjust the weight as necessary.

## PROGRAM DESCRIPTIONS

The first program, called "Gain Strength," is a foundation meant for someone who is new to strength training or has not worked out in a long time, perhaps because of a life-changing milestone, like having a baby or recovering from an injury. If you're postpartum or are coming back from injury, this is a reminder to ask your health care provider to clear you for strength training. I always recommend working with a postpartum specialist or an occupational or physical therapist before starting a new strength program.

### Gain Strength Program

The Gain Strength program, in chapter 11, is broken down into 3 different workouts per week for the first phase of 4 weeks: 1 lower body, 1 upper body, 1 total body. In weeks 5 through 8, we build up to 4 workouts per week: 1 upper body, 1 lower body, 1 upper-body push/lower-body knee dominant, 1 upper-body pull/lower-body hip dominant. Lastly, in weeks 9 through 12, there are 5 workouts per week: 1 upper body, 1 lower body, 1 upper-body push/lower-body knee dominant, 1 upper-body pull/lower-body hip dominant, 1 total body conditioning. This program can be done at home or a small gym, as long as you have dumbbells ranging from 5 to 30 pounds (2.3-13.6 kg).

## Build Sculpted Muscle Program

The Build Sculpted Muscle program, in chapter 12, is for someone who really wants to focus on getting stronger, building muscle, and having it show! These workouts emphasize fewer reps, heavy weight, and volume, volume, volume! The workouts are broken down into four different areas of focus: lower-body knee dominant, upper-body push, lower-body hip dominant, and upper-body pull. There is also an optional total body metabolic conditioning workout starting in the second phase that is recommended only if you and your body feel up to the challenge. You'll complete this program most successfully if you do it at a gym that has a barbell and rack, cable machine, bench, a 12- to 18-inch (30.48-45.72 cm) box, and a pull-up bar. If you are new to strength training, I recommend starting with the first two phases of the Gain Strength program before beginning this program.

## Get Lean Program

In chapter 13, Get Lean, the workouts are intended for someone who has strength training experience, is currently doing a workout regime or regularly attending fitness classes, and wants to pursue strength training to get lean and strong. All three phases have two workouts that emphasize heavier weights, and the other two focus on total body strength with some metabolic conditioning. Additionally, I've built in two workout days per week that consist of your favorite classes or activities—dancing, spin, Pilates, hiking, whatever! This program is perfect for someone who enjoys different types of fitness but wants to incorporate a structured strength program. I recommend you do this program at a gym that has a barbell, a squat rack, and a bench so that you are able to challenge yourself on the heavy-lifting days.

## Improve Muscle Endurance Program

The final program, Improve Muscle Endurance, in chapter 14, is ideal for someone who wants to move better, longer, and stronger. If you're someone that has a regular schedule of recreational sports, this is a great program for you. There are 4 workouts per week for 3 phases, including 1 upper body and 1 lower body, that concentrate on heavier lifting. The other two are total body workouts with a combination of strength and conditioning in multiple planes of motion. If you participate in a sport once or twice a week, you can substitute your sport for one or both of the total body workouts. As with the Get Lean program, this program can be done at home or a small gym, as long as you have a range of dumbbells from 5 to 45 pounds (2.3-20.4 kg) and a bench. As you get stronger, you may need to do this in a setting that has a barbell or weights that are heavier than 45 pounds (20.4 kg). Additionally, there are a few workouts in this program that require a cable machine, which is unlikely to be found outside a gym, but you can purchase a superband instead for use at home.

Wherever you start, it's important to keep track of your progress while training. Logging your sleep, time of day for your workout, the weights that you used, and even how you're feeling that day can help you become more aware of where you are and how far you've come over the span of the 12 weeks. I recommend using a notebook as a training log versus doing it on your phone. Unlike a phone, a notebook will not distract you every time you log your progress! I want you to be present in the time you have made for yourself. How and what you log is entirely up to you, but see figure 10.1 for a suggestion. And here's a motivation tip: write your SMART goals in your log so you can see them when you train. Plus, if you feel comfortable with the idea, I suggest filming yourself so that you can observe your form. (Note, however, that a public gym may prohibit camera use.) The more awareness you bring to your body movement, the more confident you feel. So let's get started.

# SAMPLE WORKOUT LOG

Workout Program: Workout 2, Week 1

| Exercise | Number of reps and sets | Weight (Body weight or resistance weight) | How did it feel? |
|---|---|---|---|
| **Warm-up/activation** | | | |
| 1. Rack carry | About 40 steps × 2 | 20lbs | Challenging – RPE of 5 |
| 2. Deadbug | 10 reps each side × 2 | Body weight | Easy – focused on my breath |
| 3. Side plank | 20–30 seconds each side × 2 | Body weight | Challenging right at 20 seconds |
| **Upper body** | | | |
| 4. Elevated push-up | 10 reps × 3 | Body weight | Easy! Feeling good |
| 5. Supported single-arm row | 12–15 reps each side × 3 | 20lbs | Challenging, but able to complete all reps |
| 6. Half-kneeling overhead press | 12–15 reps each side × 3 | 15lbs | Difficult, got to 12 reps |
| 7. Single-arm reverse fly | 12–15 reps each side × 3 | 5lbs | Challenging, but able to complete all reps |
| 8. Biceps curl | 12–15 reps × 3 | 10lbs | Challenging, but able to complete all reps |

**FIGURE 10.1** Sample workout log.

From B. Gozo Shimonek, *Women's Muscle & Strength* (Champaign, IL: Human Kinetics, 2025).

# 11

# GAIN STRENGTH

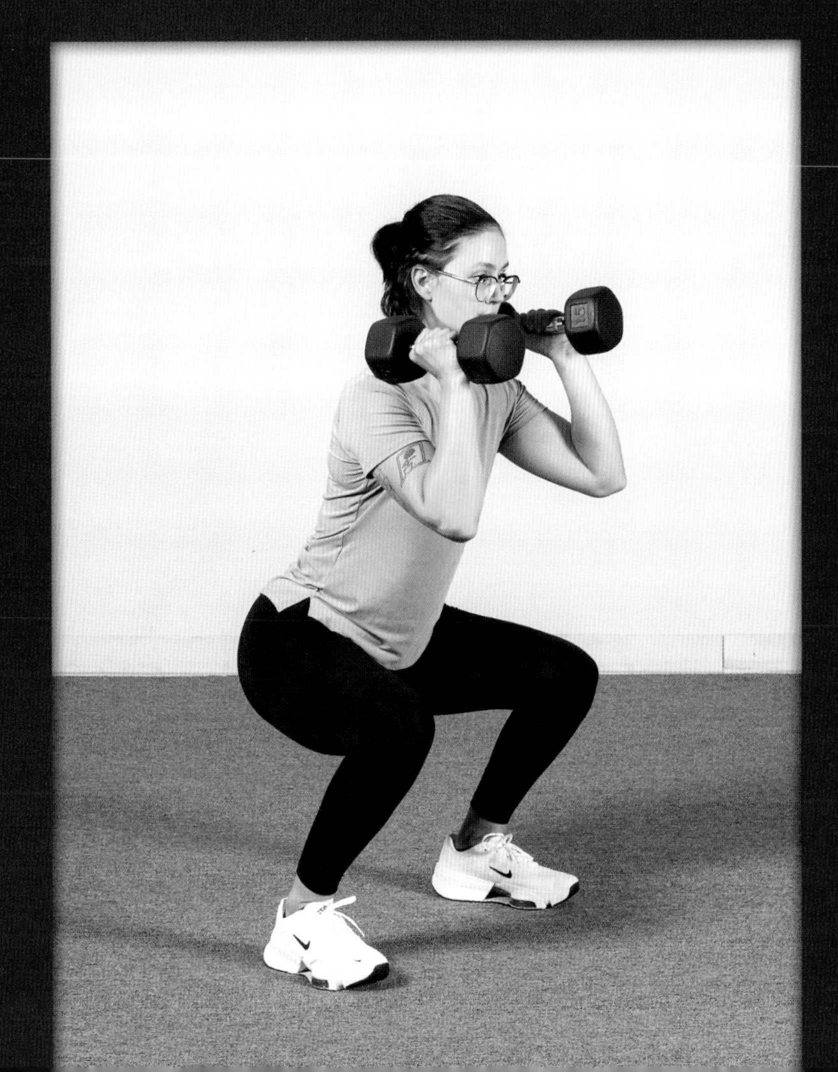

This program is designed for the beginner or for someone who has taken a long break from strength training. The program consists of many foundational strength movements, some that use body weight and some that use dumbbells. During the first four weeks of this program, you will perform 3 workouts per week: 1 lower body, 1 upper body, and 1 total body. You will build up to 4 workouts per week in weeks 5 through 8, including 1 lower body, 1 upper body, 1 upper-body push/lower-body knee dominant, and 1 upper-body pull/lower-body hip dominant. In weeks 9 through 12, you will add one more workout that includes total body conditioning. You can do this program at home or in a small gym, as long as you have dumbbells ranging from 5 to 30 pounds (2.3-13.6 kg).

Lastly, the exercises within each workout are to be performed as a circuit (i.e., back-to-back). For example, for a three-exercise workout, you'll do a set of the first exercise, then a set of the second exercise, then a set of the third exercise, and then you'll repeat this pattern for the total number of sets.

*Equipment note:* You can perform the workouts in this program with only your body weight and dumbbells. (You can add a barbell and weight plates if you'd like.)

### Gain Strength Program: Workout 1

| Exercise | Reps/time | Tempo | Sets | Exercise photo | Notes |
|---|---|---|---|---|---|
| **Weeks 1-4** | | | | | |
| **Warm-up/activation** | | | | | |
| Body-weight squat (p. 66) | 15 reps | No eccentric or isometric hold | 2 (perform as a circuit with the next 2 exercises) | | Perform with body weight only. |
| Bird dog (p. 52) | 60 sec | No eccentric or isometric hold | 2 | | |
| Body-weight reverse lunge (p. 73) | 10 reps each side | No eccentric or isometric hold | 2 | | Perform with body weight only. |

| Exercise | Reps/time | Tempo | Sets | Exercise photo | Notes |
|---|---|---|---|---|---|
| **Lower body** | | | | | |
| Goblet staggered squat (p. 70) | 12-15 reps each side | No eccentric or isometric hold | 3 (perform as a circuit with the next 3 exercises) | 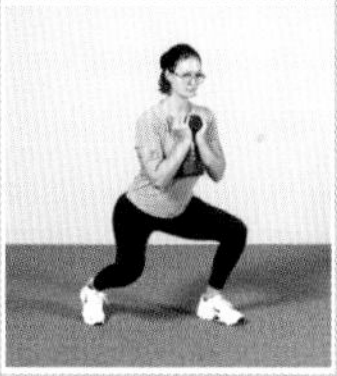 | |
| Romanian deadlift (p. 85) | 12-15 reps | No eccentric or isometric hold | 3 | 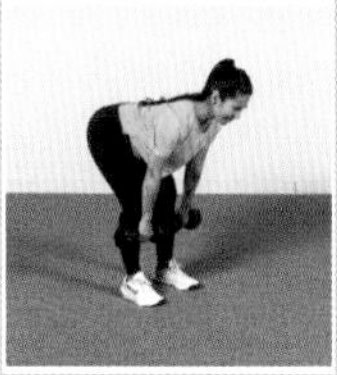 | |
| Dumbbell reverse lunge (p. 73) | 12-15 reps each side | No eccentric or isometric hold | 3 | 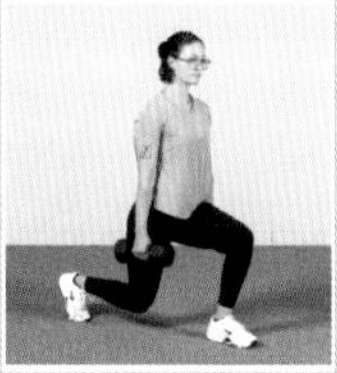 | |
| Barbell or body-weight hip thrust (p. 83) | 12-15 reps | 1, 3, 3 | 3 | 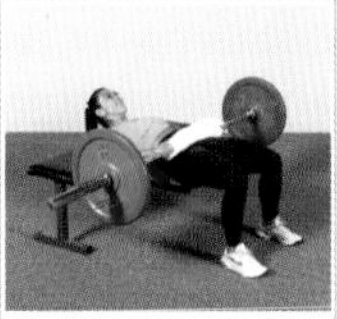 | Start with body weight. |
| **Weeks 5-8** | | | | | |
| **Warm-up/activation** | | | | | |
| Body-weight squat (p. 66) | 15 reps | 3, 1, 1 | 2 (perform as a circuit with the next 2 exercises) | 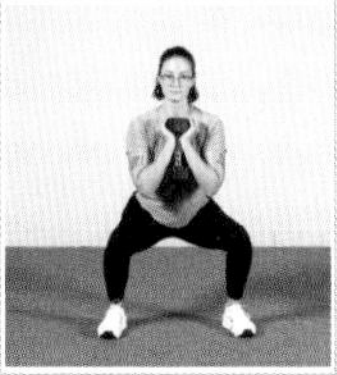 | Perform with body weight only. |
| Bird dog (p. 52) | 60 sec | No eccentric or isometric hold | 2 | 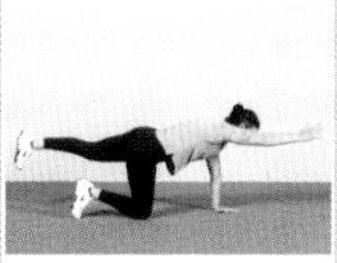 | |
| Body-weight reverse lunge (p. 73) | 10 reps each side | No eccentric or isometric hold | 2 | 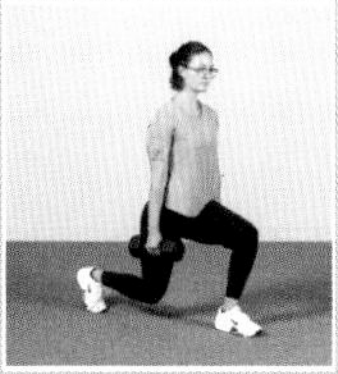 | Perform with body weight only. |

*(continued)*

## Gain Strength Program: Workout 1 *(continued)*

| Exercise | Reps/time | Tempo | Sets | Exercise photo | Notes |
|---|---|---|---|---|---|
| **Lower body** | | | | | |
| Goblet squat (p. 66) | 10-12 reps | No eccentric or isometric hold | 3 (perform as a circuit with the next 3 exercises) | 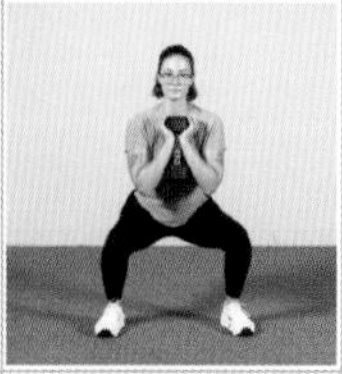 | |
| Romanian deadlift (p. 85) | 10-12 reps | 5, 1, 1 | 3 | 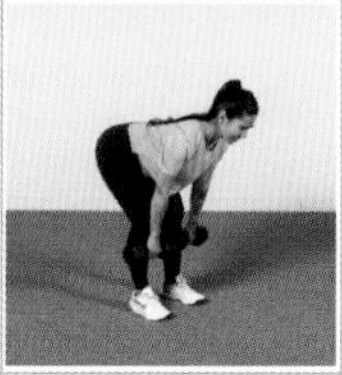 | |
| Alternating goblet dumbbell reverse lunge (p. 73) | 10-12 reps each side | No eccentric or isometric hold | 3 | 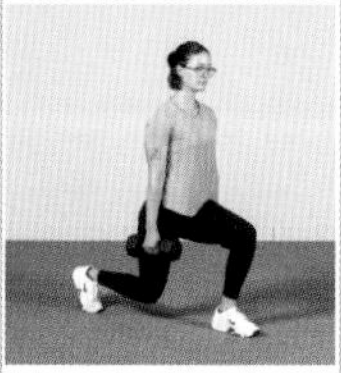 | Use goblet grip. |
| Barbell or dumbbell hip thrust (p. 83) | 12-15 reps | 1, 3, 3 | 3 | 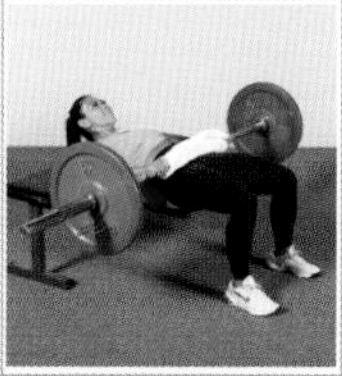 | Start with dumbbells. |
| **Weeks 9-12** | | | | | |
| **Warm-up/activation** | | | | | |
| Body-weight squat (p. 66) | 15 reps | No eccentric or isometric hold | 2 (perform as a circuit with the next 2 exercises | 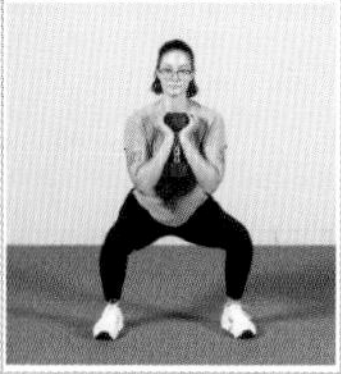 | Perform with body weight only. |
| Bird dog (p. 52) | 60 sec | No eccentric or isometric hold | 2 | 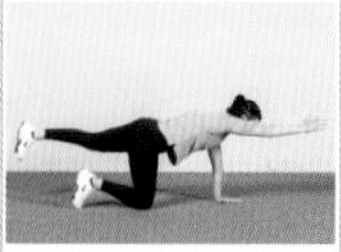 | |
| Body-weight reverse lunge (p. 73) | 10 reps each side | No eccentric or isometric hold | 2 | 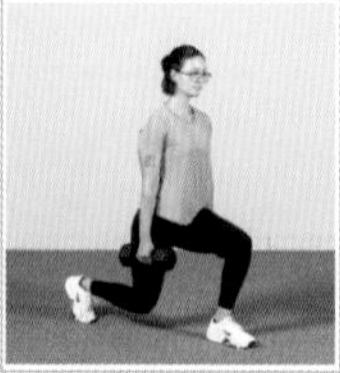 | Perform with body weight only. |

| Exercise | Reps/time | Tempo | Sets | Exercise photo | Notes |
|---|---|---|---|---|---|
| **Lower body** | | | | | |
| Front rack dumbbell squat (p. 66) | 8-10 reps | No eccentric or isometric hold | 3 (perform as a circuit with the next 5 exercises) | 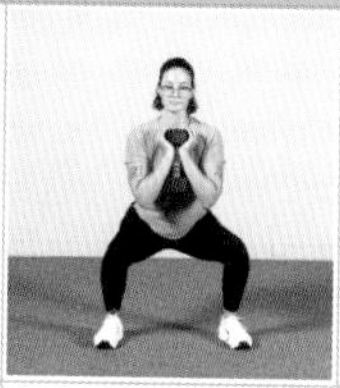 | Use rack position. |
| Barbell or dumbbell hip thrust (p. 83) | 10-12 reps | No eccentric or isometric hold | 3 | 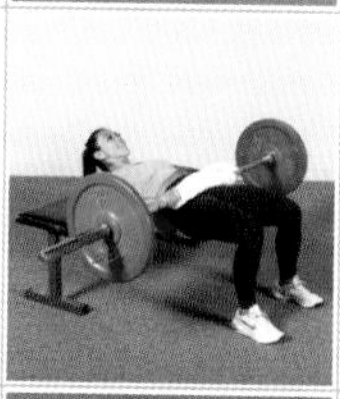 | Start with dumbbells. |
| Side-lying hip circles (p. 92) | 15 reps each direction on each side | No eccentric or isometric hold | 3 | 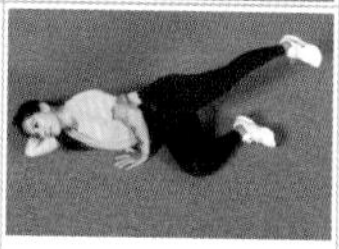 | |
| Rest 90 sec to 3 min as needed | | | | | |
| Alternating goblet forward lunge (p. 74) | 8-10 reps each side | No eccentric or isometric hold | 3 | 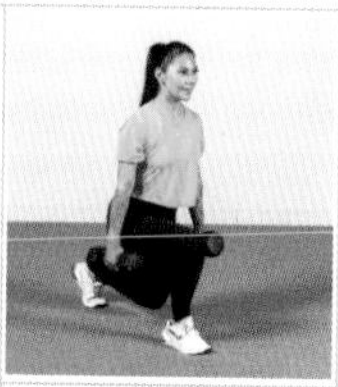 | Use goblet grip. |
| Romanian deadlift (p. 85) | 8-10 reps | 5, 1, 1 | 3 | 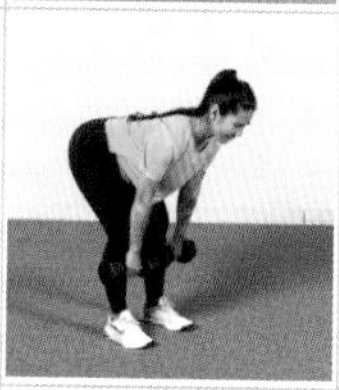 | |
| Staggered bridge (p. 82) | 15 reps each side | 1, 3, 3 | 3 | 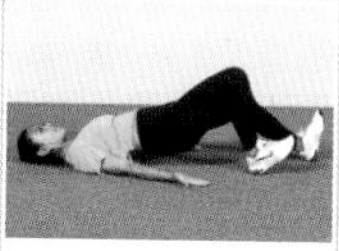 | |

## Gain Strength Program: Workout 2

| Exercise | Reps/time | Tempo | Sets | Exercise photo | Notes |
|---|---|---|---|---|---|
| | | Weeks 1-4 | | | |
| | | Warm-up/activation | | | |
| Rack carry (p. 45) | About 40 steps | No eccentric or isometric hold | 2 (perform as a circuit with the next 2 exercises) | | |
| Deadbug (p. 54) | 10 reps each side | No eccentric or isometric hold | 2 | | |
| High side plank (p. 56) | 20-30 sec each side | No eccentric or isometric hold | 2 | | |
| | | Upper body | | | |
| Elevated push-up (p. 99) | 10 reps | 3, 1, 1 | 3 (perform as a circuit with the next 5 exercises) | | |
| Supported single-arm row (p. 119) | 12-15 reps each side | 1, 1, 3 | 3 | | |
| Dumbbell bent-over row (p. 118) | 12-15 reps | 3, 1, 1 | 3 | | |

| Exercise | Reps/time | Tempo | Sets | Exercise photo | Notes |
|---|---|---|---|---|---|
| Half-kneeling overhead press (p. 106) | 12-15 reps each side | 1, 1, 3 | 3 | | |
| Single-arm reverse fly (p. 121) | 12-15 reps each side | No eccentric or isometric hold | 3 | | Perform with single arm. |
| Dumbbell biceps curl (p. 124) | 12-15 reps | No eccentric or isometric hold | 3 | | |
| **Weeks 5-8** | | | | | |
| **Warm-up/activation** | | | | | |
| Rack carry (p. 45) | About 40 steps | No eccentric or isometric hold | 2 (perform as a circuit with the next 2 exercises) | | |
| Deadbug (p. 54) | 10 reps each side | No eccentric or isometric hold | 2 | | |
| Forearm side plank (p. 56) | 20-30 sec each side | No eccentric or isometric hold | 2 | | |

*(continued)*

## Gain Strength Program: Workout 2 *(continued)*

| Exercise | Reps/time | Tempo | Sets | Exercise photo | Notes |
|---|---|---|---|---|---|
| | | **Upper body** | | | |
| Alternating dumbbell floor press (p. 102) | 10-12 reps each side | 1, 1, 3 | 3 (perform as a circuit with the next 4 exercises) | | Perform as alternating. |
| Alternating dumbbell bent-over row (p. 118) | 10-12 reps each side (rest halfway if needed) | 1, 1, 3 | 3 | | Perform as alternating. |
| Alternating tall kneeling overhead press (p. 107) | 10-12 reps each side | 1, 1, 3 | 3 | | Perform as alternating. |
| Rest 90 sec to 3 min as needed | | | | | |
| Lying triceps extension (p. 114) | 12-15 reps | No eccentric or isometric hold | 3 | | |
| Dumbbell biceps curl (p. 124) | 12-15 reps | No eccentric or isometric hold | 3 | | |

| Exercise | Reps/time | Tempo | Sets | Exercise photo | Notes |
|---|---|---|---|---|---|
| **Weeks 9-12** | | | | | |
| **Warm-up/activation** | | | | | |
| Rack carry (p. 45) | About 40 steps | No eccentric or isometric hold | 2 (perform as a circuit with the next 2 exercises) | 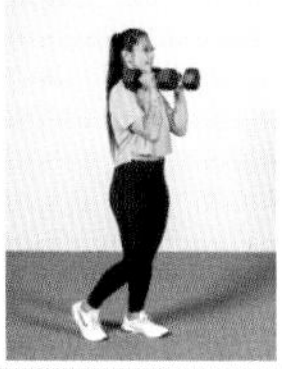 | |
| Deadbug (p. 54) | 10 reps each side | No eccentric or isometric hold | 2 | 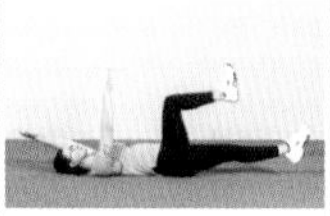 | |
| Forearm side plank (p. 56) | 20-30 sec each side | No eccentric or isometric hold | 2 | 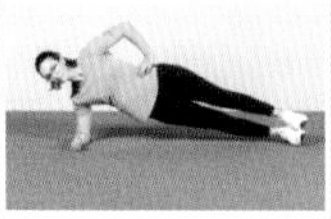 | |
| **Upper body** | | | | | |
| Dumbbell floor press (p. 102) | 8-10 reps | 1, 1, 3 | 3 (perform as a circuit with the next 4 exercises) | 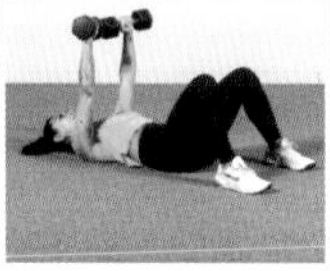 | |
| Dumbbell bent-over row (p. 118) | 10-12 reps | 1, 1, 3 | 3 | 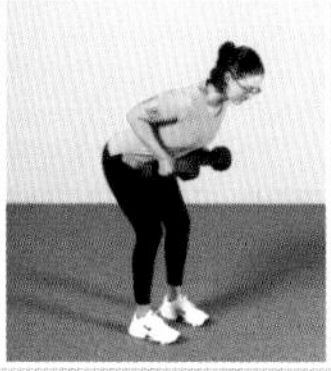 | |
| Tall kneeling overhead press (p. 107) | 8-10 reps | 1, 1, 3 | 3 | 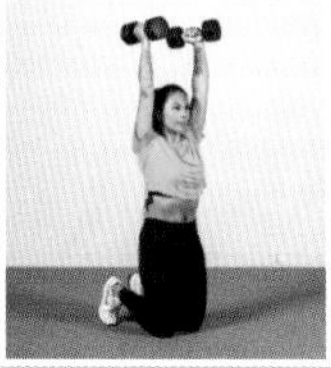 | |
| Reverse fly (p. 121) | 8-10 reps | No eccentric or isometric hold | 3 | 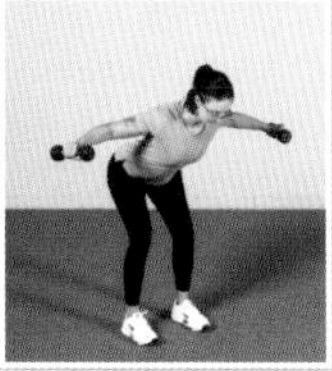 | |
| Lying triceps extension (p. 114) | 8-10 reps | No eccentric or isometric hold | 3 | 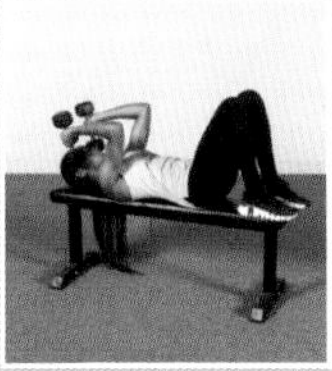 | |

## Gain Strength Program: Workout 3

| Exercise | Reps/time | Tempo | Sets | Exercise photo | Notes |
|---|---|---|---|---|---|
| **Weeks 1-4** | | | | | |
| **Warm-up/activation** | | | | | |
| Deadbug (p. 54) | 10 reps each side | No eccentric or isometric hold | 2 (perform as a circuit with the next 3 exercises) | | |
| Shoulder tap (p. 59) | 10 reps each side | No eccentric or isometric hold | 2 | | |
| Bridge (p. 81) | 10 reps | 1, 3, 3 | 2 | | |
| Suitcase carry (p. 44) | About 20 steps each side | No eccentric or isometric hold | 2 | | |
| **Total body** | | | | | |
| Dumbbell push press (p. 109) | 6-8 reps | X, 1, 5 | 3 (perform as a circuit with the next 3 exercises) | | |
| Dumbbell Bulgarian split squat (p. 76) | 6-8 reps each side | 5, 1, 1 | 3 | | |
| Dumbbell hammer curl (p. 125) | 8-10 reps | 1, 1, 5 | 3 | | |
| Romanian deadlift (p. 85) | 8-10 reps | 5, 3, 1 | 3 | | |

| Exercise | Reps/time | Tempo | Sets | Exercise photo | Notes |
|---|---|---|---|---|---|
| **Weeks 5-8** | | | | | |
| **Warm-up/activation** | | | | | |
| Deadbug (p. 54) | 10 reps each side | No eccentric or isometric hold | 2 (perform as a circuit with the next 3 exercises) | | |
| Shoulder tap (p. 59) | 10 reps each side | No eccentric or isometric hold | 2 | | |
| Bridge (p. 81) | 10 reps | 1, 3, 3 | 2 | | |
| Suitcase carry (p. 44) | About 20 steps each side | No eccentric or isometric hold | 2 | | |
| **Upper-body push/lower-body knee dominant** | | | | | |
| Push-up *or* elevated or wall push-up (p. 99) | 6-8 reps | 1, 5, 1 | 3 (perform as a circuit with the next 3 exercises) | | |
| Dumbbell Bulgarian split squat (p. 76) | 6-8 reps each side | 1, 5, 1 | 3 | | |
| Rotational overhead press (p. 140) | 8-10 reps each side | No eccentric or isometric hold | 3 | | |
| Goblet sumo squat (p. 71) | 8-10 reps | 1, 5, 1 | 3 | | |

(continued)

## Gain Strength Program: Workout 3 *(continued)*

| Exercise | Reps/time | Tempo | Sets | Exercise photo | Notes |
|---|---|---|---|---|---|
| **Weeks 9-12** | | | | | |
| **Warm-up/activation** | | | | | |
| Deadbug (p. 54) | 10 reps each side | No eccentric or isometric hold | 2 (perform as a circuit with the next 3 exercises) | | |
| Shoulder tap (p. 59) | 10 reps each side | No eccentric or isometric hold | 2 | | |
| Bridge (p. 81) | 10 reps | 1, 3, 3 | 2 | | |
| Suitcase carry (p. 44) | About 20 steps each side | No eccentric or isometric hold | 2 | | |
| **Upper-body push/lower-body knee dominant** | | | | | |
| Push-up *or* elevated or wall push-up (p. 99) | 6-8 reps | 5, 5, 1 | 3 (perform as a circuit with the next 3 exercises) | | |
| Dumbbell Bulgarian split squat (p. 76) | 6-8 reps each side | 5, 5, 1 | 3 | | |
| Rotational overhead press (p. 140) | 6-8 reps each side | No eccentric or isometric hold | 3 | | |
| Goblet sumo squat (p. 71) | 8-10 reps | 5, 5, 1 | 3 | | |

## Gain Strength Program: Workout 4

Start adding a fourth workout in week 5 of the program.

| Exercise | Reps/time | Tempo | Sets | Exercise photo | Notes |
|---|---|---|---|---|---|
| Weeks 5-8 | | | | | |
| **Warm-up/activation** | | | | | |
| High goblet carry (p. 46) | About 40 steps | No eccentric or isometric hold | 2 (perform as a circuit with the next 3 exercises) | 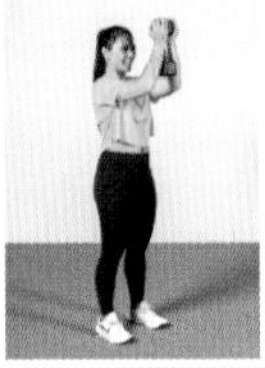 | |
| Prone back extension (p. 148) | 15 reps | No eccentric or isometric hold | 2 | 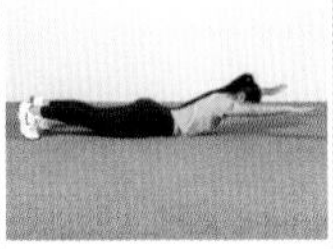 | |
| Body-weight hip thrust (p. 83) | 15 reps | 1, 5, 1 | 2 | 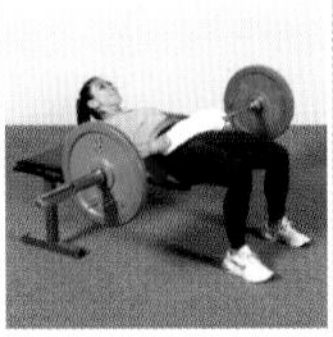 | Perform with body weight only. |
| Hollow hold (p. 60) | 15-20 sec | No eccentric or isometric hold | 2 | 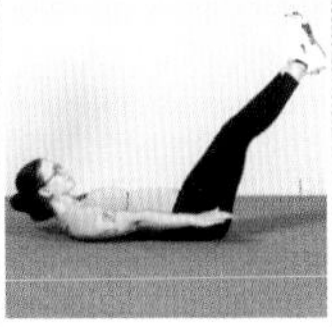 | |
| **Upper-body pull/lower-body hip dominant** | | | | | |
| Dumbbell bent-over row (p. 118) | 10-12 reps | 1, 5, 1 | 3 (perform as a circuit with the next 3 exercises) | 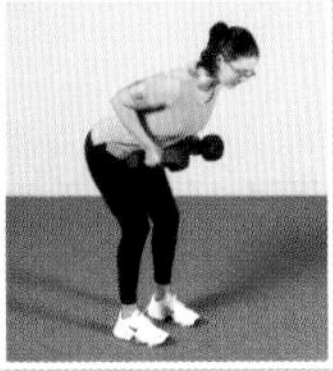 | Reset after each rep if necessary. |
| Staggered barbell or body-weight hip thrust (p. 84) | 8-10 reps each side | 1, 3, 5 | 3 | 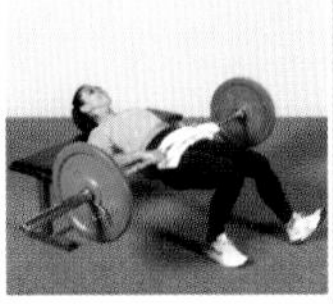 | Start with body weight. |
| Single-arm reverse fly on a bench (p. 121) | 8-10 reps each side | 1, 1, 5 | 3 | 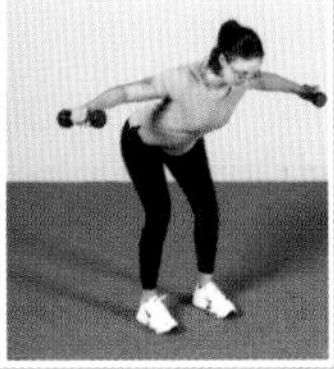 | Perform on bench with single arm; see reverse fly for mechanics. |

*(continued)*

## Gain Strength Program: Workout 4 *(continued)*

| Exercise | Reps/time | Tempo | Sets | Exercise photo | Notes |
|---|---|---|---|---|---|
| Staggered Romanian dead-lift (p. 86) | 10-12 reps each side | 5, 3, 1 | 3 | | |
| **Weeks 9-12** | | | | | |
| **Warm-up/activation** | | | | | |
| High goblet carry (p. 46) | About 40 steps | No eccentric or isometric hold | 2 (perform as a circuit with the next 3 exercises) | | |
| Prone back extension (p. 148) | 15 reps | No eccentric or isometric hold | 2 | | |
| Body-weight hip thrust (p. 83) | 15 reps | 1, 5, 1 | 2 | | Perform with body weight only. |
| Hollow hold (p. 60) | 15-20 sec | No eccentric or isometric hold | 2 | | |
| **Upper-body pull/lower-body hip dominant** | | | | | |
| Dumbbell bent-over row (p. 118) | 8-10 reps | 1, 5, 5 | 3 (perform as a circuit with the next 3 exercises) | | Reset after each rep if necessary. |
| Single-leg bridge (p. 82) | 10-12 reps each side | 1, 5, 5 | 3 | | |

| Exercise | Reps/time | Tempo | Sets | Exercise photo | Notes |
|---|---|---|---|---|---|
| Single-arm reverse fly on a bench (p. 121) | 8-10 reps each side | 1, 1, 5 | 3 | | Perform on bench with single arm; see reverse fly for mechanics. |
| Staggered Romanian dead-lift (p. 86) | 8-10 reps each side | 5, 1, 1 | 3 | | |

## Gain Strength Program: Workout 5

Start adding a fifth workout in week 9 of the program.

| Exercise | Reps/time | Tempo | Sets | Exercise photo | Notes |
|---|---|---|---|---|---|
| **Weeks 9-12** | | | | | |
| **Warm-up/activation** | | | | | |
| Farmer carry (p. 43) | About 40 steps | No eccentric or isometric hold | 2 (perform as a circuit with the next 3 exercises) | | |
| High plank (p. 58) | 30-45 sec | No eccentric or isometric hold | 2 | | |
| Side plank leg lift (p. 57) | 10 reps each side | No eccentric or isometric hold | 2 | | |
| Prone W back extension (p. 149) | 15 reps | No eccentric or isometric hold | 2 | | |

*(continued)*

## Gain Strength Program: Workout 5 *(continued)*

| Exercise | Reps/time | Tempo | Sets | Exercise photo | Notes |
|---|---|---|---|---|---|
| **Total body conditioning** | | | | | |
| Alternating plank row (p. 142) | 10-12 reps each side | No eccentric or isometric hold | 3 (perform as a circuit with the next 3 exercises) | | |
| Half-kneeling dynamic low to high lift (p. 138) | 10-12 reps each side | X, X, 3 | 3 | | |
| Hinge to row rotation (p. 144) | 10-12 reps each side | No eccentric or isometric hold | 3 | | |
| Squat to overhead press (p. 143) | 10-12 reps | No eccentric or isometric hold | 3 | | |

12

# BUILD SCULPTED MUSCLE

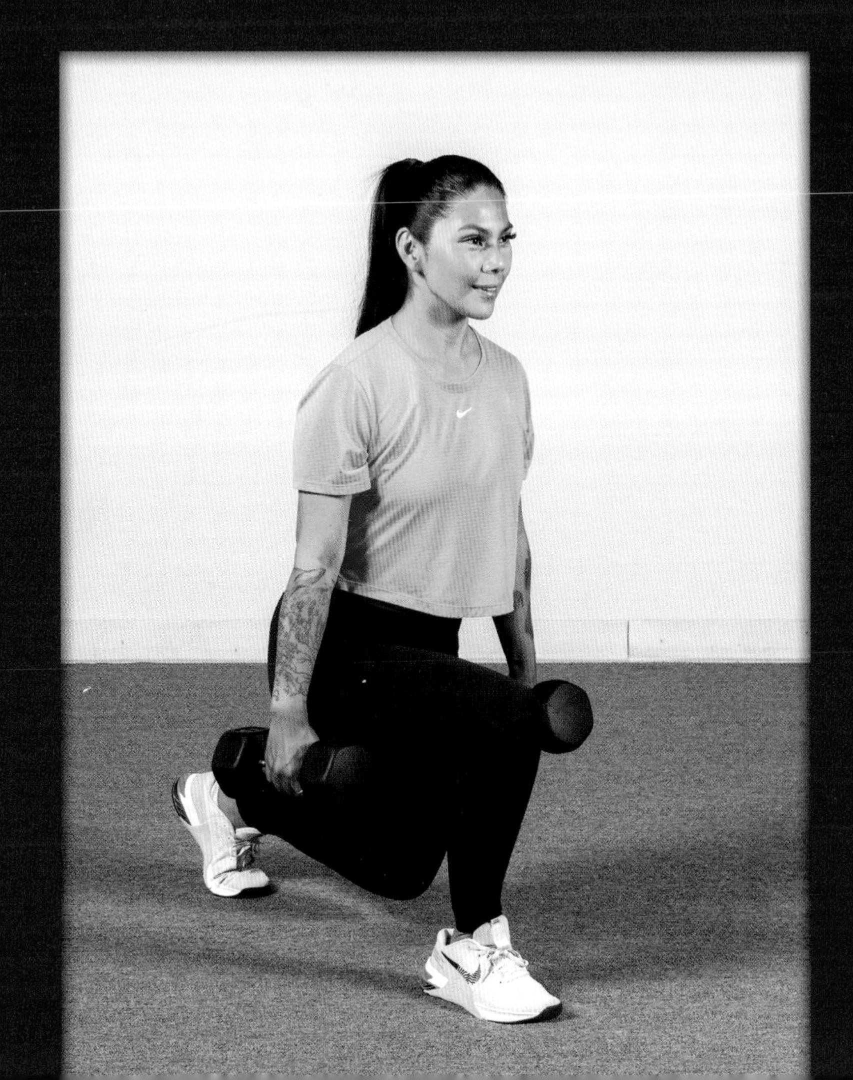

This program is ideal for someone who has already done some strength training but wants a program specifically for sculpting muscles. The workouts focus on a lower rep range with a heavy weight, which adds up to a *lot* of volume. The workouts are divided into four categories: lower-body knee dominant, upper-body push, lower-body hip dominant, and upper-body pull. The second phase starts in weeks 5-8 and adds an optional metabolic conditioning workout. Throughout the program, you'll want to perform the exercises within each workout as a circuit (i.e., back-to-back).

*Equipment note:* The workouts in this program require a fully equipped gym with access to a barbell and squat rack, a cable machine, a bench, a variety of dumbbells, a 12- to 18-inch (30.48-45.72 cm) box, and a pull-up bar.

### Build Sculpted Muscle Program: Workout 1

| Exercise | Reps/time | Tempo | Sets | Exercise photo | Notes |
|---|---|---|---|---|---|
| **Weeks 1-4** | | | | | |
| **Warm-up/activation** | | | | | |
| Deadbug (p. 54) | 10 reps each side | No eccentric or isometric hold | 2 (perform as a circuit with the next 3 exercises) | | |
| Body-weight squat (p. 66) | 10 reps | 3, 1, 1 | 2 | | Perform with body weight only. |
| Farmer carry (p. 43) | About 40 steps | No eccentric or isometric hold | 2 | | |
| Body-weight stationary lunge or split squat (p. 75) | 10 reps each side | No eccentric or isometric hold | 2 | | Perform with body weight only. |

| Exercise | Reps/time | Tempo | Sets | Exercise photo | Notes |
|---|---|---|---|---|---|
| **Lower-body knee dominant** | | | | | |
| Front rack squat with dumbbells or barbell (p. 68) | 6-8 reps | 5, 1, 1 | 5 with 2 min rest between sets | | |
| Alternating dumbbell reverse lunge (p. 73) | 10-12 reps each side | No eccentric or isometric hold | 4 (perform as a circuit with the next 2 exercises) | | |
| Goblet stationary lateral lunge (p. 78) | 10-12 reps each side | No eccentric or isometric hold | 4 | | Use goblet grip. |
| Wall sit (p. 72) | 30-45 sec | No eccentric or isometric hold | 4 | | |
| **Weeks 5-8** | | | | | |
| **Warm-up/activation** | | | | | |
| Deadbug (p. 54) | 10 reps each side | No eccentric or isometric hold | 2 (perform as a circuit with the next 3 exercises) | | |
| Body-weight squat (p. 66) | 10 reps | 3, 1, 1 | 2 | | Perform with body weight only. |
| Farmer carry (p. 43) | About 40 steps | No eccentric or isometric hold | 2 | | |
| Body-weight stationary lateral lunge (p. 78) | 10 reps each side | No eccentric or isometric hold | 2 | | Perform with body weight only. |

*(continued)*

## Build Sculpted Muscle Program: Workout 1 *(continued)*

| Exercise | Reps/time | Tempo | Sets | Exercise photo | Notes |
|---|---|---|---|---|---|
| **Lower-body knee dominant** | | | | | |
| Front rack squat with dumbbells or barbell (p. 68) | 6-8 reps | 5, 5, 1 | 5 with 2 min rest between sets | | |
| Dumbbell lateral lunge (p. 78) | 10-12 reps each side | No eccentric or isometric hold | 4 (perform as a circuit with the next 2 exer-cises) | | |
| Goblet sumo squat (p. 71) | 8-10 reps | 1, 5, 1 | 4 | | |
| Dumbbell step-up (p. 77) | 10-12 reps each side | No eccentric or isometric hold | 4 | | |
| **Weeks 9-12** | | | | | |
| **Warm-up/activation** | | | | | |
| Deadbug (p. 54) | 10 reps each side | | 2 (perform as a circuit with the next 3 exer-cises) | | |
| Body-weight squat (p. 66) | 10 reps | 3, 1, 1 | 2 | | Perform with body weight only. |
| Farmer carry (p. 43) | About 40 steps | No eccentric or isometric hold | 2 | | |
| Body-weight stationary lateral lunge (p. 78) | 10 reps each side | No eccentric or isometric hold | 2 | | Perform with body weight only. |

| Exercise | Reps/time | Tempo | Sets | Exercise photo | Notes |
|---|---|---|---|---|---|
| **Lower-body knee dominant** | | | | | |
| Barbell back squat (p. 67) | 6-8 reps | No eccentric or isometric hold | 5 with 2 minutes rest between sets | | |
| Staggered front rack dumbbell squat (p. 70) | 8-10 reps each side | 3, 1, 1 | 4 (perform as a circuit with the next 2 exercises) | | Use front rack position. |
| Dumbbell forward lunge (p. 74) | 8-10 reps each side | No eccentric or isometric hold | 4 | | |
| Goblet back diagonal lunge (p. 80) | 10-12 reps each side | No eccentric or isometric hold | 4 | | Use goblet grip. |

## Build Sculpted Muscle Program: Workout 2

| Exercise | Reps/time | Tempo | Sets | Exercise photo | Notes |
|---|---|---|---|---|---|
| **Weeks 1-4** | | | | | |
| **Warm-up/activation** | | | | | |
| High plank (p. 58) | 30-45 sec | No eccentric or isometric hold | 2 (perform as a circuit with the next 3 exercises) | | |
| Half-kneeling Paloff press (p. 51) | 10 reps each side | 1, 3, 3 | 2 | | |
| Dead hang (p. 48) | 15-30 sec | No eccentric or isometric hold | 2 | | |

(continued)

## Build Sculpted Muscle Program: Workout 2 *(continued)*

| Exercise | Reps/time | Tempo | Sets | Exercise photo | Notes |
|---|---|---|---|---|---|
| Suitcase carry (p. 44) | About 20 steps each side | No eccentric or isometric hold | 2 | | |
| **Upper-body push** | | | | | |
| Dumbbell or barbell chest press (p. 100) | 6-8 reps | 1, 1, 5 | 5 with 2 min rest between sets | | |
| Half-kneeling overhead press (p. 106) | 10-12 reps each side | 1, 1, 3 | 4 (perform as a circuit with the next 3 exercises) | | |
| Dumbbell lateral raise (p. 112) | 10-12 reps | No eccentric or isometric hold | 4 | | |
| Push-up *or* elevated or wall push-up (p. 99) | 10-12 reps | 3, 1, 1 | 4 | | |
| Lying triceps extension (p. 114) | 10-12 reps | No eccentric or isometric hold | 4 | | |
| **Weeks 5-8** | | | | | |
| **Warm-up/activation** | | | | | |
| High plank (p. 58) | 30-45 sec | No eccentric or isometric hold | 2 (perform as a circuit with the next 3 exercises) | | |
| Half-kneeling Paloff press (p. 51) | 10 reps each side | 1, 3, 3 | 2 | | |

| Exercise | Reps/time | Tempo | Sets | Exercise photo | Notes |
|---|---|---|---|---|---|
| Dead hang (p. 48) | 15-30 sec | No eccentric or isometric hold | 2 | | |
| Suitcase carry (p. 44) | About 20 steps each side | No eccentric or isometric hold | 2 | | |
| **Upper-body push** | | | | | |
| Dumbbell or barbell chest press (p. 100) | 6-8 reps | 1, 5, 5 | 5 with 2 min rest in between sets | | |
| Alternating dumbbell push press (p. 109) | 10-12 reps each side | No eccentric or isometric hold | 4 (perform as a circuit with the next 3 exercises) | | Perform as alternating. |
| Alternating cable chest fly (p. 105) | 10-12 reps each side | 1, 1, 3 | 4 | | Perform as alternating. |
| Dumbbell Arnold press (p. 110) | 10-12 reps | No eccentric or isometric hold | 4 | | |
| Triceps kickback (p. 113) | 10-12 reps | No eccentric or isometric hold | 4 | | |

*(continued)*

## Build Sculpted Muscle Program: Workout 2 *(continued)*

| Exercise | Reps/time | Tempo | Sets | Exercise photo | Notes |
|---|---|---|---|---|---|
| **Weeks 9-12** | | | | | |
| **Warm-up/activation** | | | | | |
| High plank (p. 58) | 30-45 sec | No eccentric or isometric hold | 2 (perform as a circuit with the next 3 exercises) | | |
| Half-kneeling Paloff press (p. 51) | 10 reps each side | 1, 3, 3 | 2 | | |
| Dead hang (p. 48) | 15-30 sec | No eccentric or isometric hold | 2 | | |
| Suitcase carry (p. 44) | About 20 steps each side | No eccentric or isometric hold | 2 | | |
| **Upper-body push** | | | | | |
| Push-up *or* elevated or wall push-up (p. 99) | 6-8 reps | 5, 1, 1 | 5 (perform as a superset with the next exercise, resting 2 min between rounds) | | |
| Dumbbell or barbell chest press (p. 100) | 6-8 reps | No eccentric or isometric hold | 5 | | |

| Exercise | Reps/time | Tempo | Sets | Exercise photo | Notes |
|---|---|---|---|---|---|
| Dumbbell push press (p. 109) | 10-12 reps | No eccentric or isometric hold | 4 (perform as a circuit with the next 3 exer-cises) | 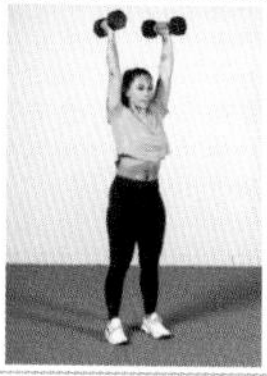 | |
| Cable chest fly (p. 105) | 10-12 reps | No eccentric or isometric hold | 4 | 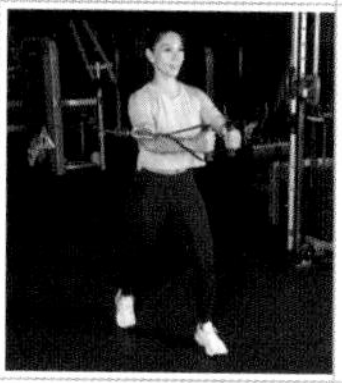 | |
| Dumbbell front raise (p. 111) | 10-12 reps | No eccentric or isometric hold | 4 | 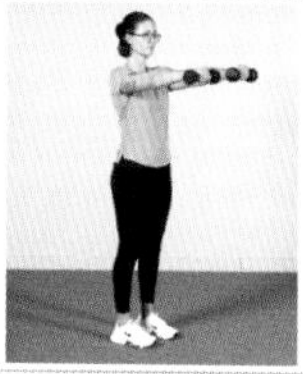 | |
| Dumbbell lateral raise (p. 112) | 10-12 reps | No eccentric or isometric hold | 4 | 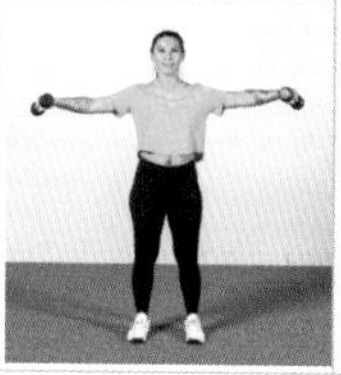 | |

## Build Sculpted Muscle Program: Workout 3

| Exercise | Reps/time | Tempo | Sets | Exercise photo | Notes |
|---|---|---|---|---|---|
| | | Weeks 1-4 | | | |
| | | Warm-up/activation | | | |
| Deadbug (p. 54) | 10 reps each side | No eccentric or isometric hold | 2 (perform as a circuit with the next 3 exercises) | | |
| Shoulder tap (p. 59) | 10 reps each side | No eccentric or isometric hold | 2 | | |
| Bridge (p. 81) | 15 reps | 1, 3, 1 | 2 | | |
| Farmer carry (p. 43) | About 40 steps | No eccentric or isometric hold | 2 | | |
| | | Lower-body hip dominant | | | |
| Barbell hip thrust (p. 83) | 6-8 reps | 1, 1, 5 | 5 with 2 min rest between sets | | |
| Romanian deadlift (p. 85) | 8-10 reps | 5, 1, 1 | 4 (perform as a circuit with the next 2 exercises) | | |
| Cable kickback (p. 94) | 8-10 reps each side | No eccentric or isometric hold | 4 | | |
| Side-lying abduction (p. 93) | 15 reps each side | No eccentric or isometric hold | 4 | | |

| Exercise | Reps/time | Tempo | Sets | Exercise photo | Notes |
|---|---|---|---|---|---|
| **Weeks 5-8** | | | | | |
| **Warm-up/activation** | | | | | |
| Deadbug (p. 54) | 10 reps each side | No eccentric or isometric hold | 2 (perform as a circuit with the next 3 exercises) | | |
| Shoulder tap (p. 59) | 10 reps each side | No eccentric or isometric hold | 2 | | |
| Bridge (p. 81) | 15 reps | 1, 3, 1 | 2 | | |
| Farmer carry (p. 43) | About 40 steps | No eccentric or isometric hold | 2 | | |
| **Lower-body hip dominant** | | | | | |
| Barbell hip thrust (p. 83) | 6-8 reps | 1, 5, 5 | 5 with 2 min rest between sets | | |
| Staggered Romanian deadlift (p. 86) | 8-10 reps each side | 3, 1, 1 | 4 (perform as a circuit with the next 2 exercises) | | |
| Barbell good morning (p. 88) | 8-10 reps | 3, 1, 1 | 4 | | |
| Cable abduction (p. 95) | 15 reps each side | No eccentric or isometric hold | 4 | | |

*(continued)*

## Build Sculpted Muscle Program: Workout 3 *(continued)*

| Exercise | Reps/time | Tempo | Sets | Exercise photo | Notes |
|---|---|---|---|---|---|
| | | **Weeks 9-12** | | | |
| | | **Warm-up/activation** | | | |
| Deadbug (p. 54) | 10 reps each side | No eccentric or isometric hold | 2 (perform as a circuit with the next 3 exercises) | | |
| Shoulder tap (p. 59) | 10 reps each side | No eccentric or isometric hold | 2 | | |
| Bridge (p. 81) | 15 reps | 1, 3, 1 | 2 | | |
| Farmer carry (p. 43) | About 40 steps | No eccentric or isometric hold | 2 | | |
| | | **Lower-body hip dominant** | | | |
| Barbell or body-weight good morning (p. 88) | 10-12 reps | 3, 1, 1 | 5 (perform as a superset with the next exercise, resting 2 min between rounds) | | Start with body weight. |
| Conventional or American deadlift (p. 89) | 6-8 reps | No eccentric or isometric hold | 5 | | |

| Exercise | Reps/time | Tempo | Sets | Exercise photo | Notes |
|---|---|---|---|---|---|
| Staggered hip thrust with barbell or dumbbells (p. 84) | 8-10 reps each side | 1, 3, 1 | 4 (perform as a circuit with the next 2 exercises) | 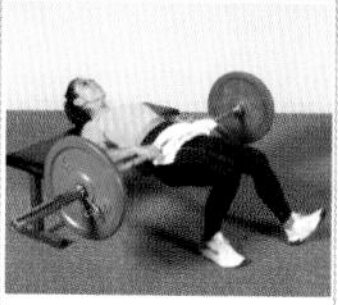 | |
| Long bridge (p. 82) | 10-12 reps | 1, 3, 1 | 4 | 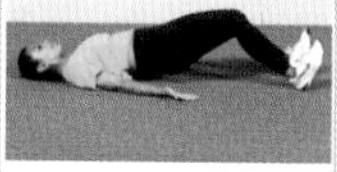 | |
| Side-lying hip circles (p. 92) | 15 reps each direction and each side | No eccentric or isometric hold | 4 | 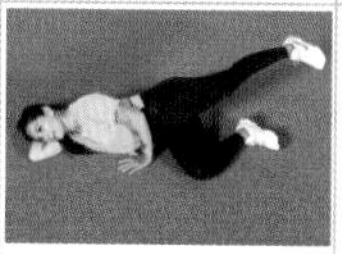 | |

## Build Sculpted Muscle Program: Workout 4

| Exercise | Reps/time | Tempo | Sets | Exercise photo | Notes |
|---|---|---|---|---|---|
| **Weeks 1-4** | | | | | |
| **Warm-up/activation** | | | | | |
| Deadbug (p. 54) | 10 reps each side | No eccentric or isometric hold | 2 (perform as a circuit with the next 3 exercises) | 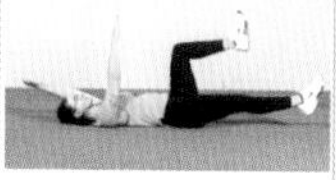 | |
| High goblet carry (p. 46) | About 40 steps | No eccentric or isometric hold | 2 | 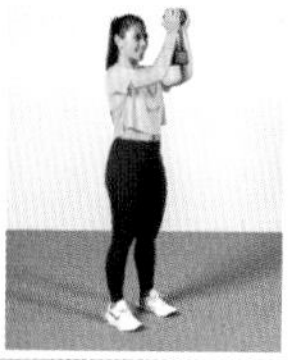 | |
| Active hang (p. 49) | 15-30 sec | No eccentric or isometric hold | 2 | 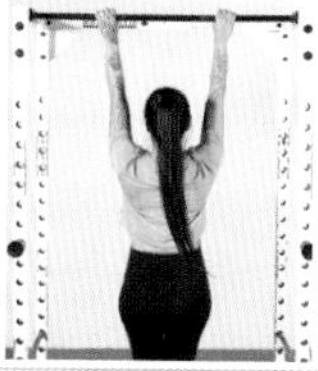 | |
| Prone back extension (p. 148) | 15 reps | No eccentric or isometric hold | 2 | 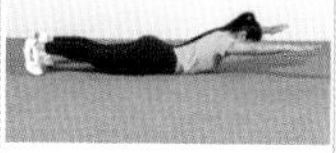 | |

(continued)

## Build Sculpted Muscle Program: Workout 4 *(continued)*

| Exercise | Reps/time | Tempo | Sets | Exercise photo | Notes |
|---|---|---|---|---|---|
| **Upper-body pull** | | | | | |
| Neutral or supinated grip pull-up/chin-up (p. 127) | 5-8 reps (or max reps) | Max isometric hold | 5 (perform as a superset with the next exercise, resting 2 min between rounds) | | |
| Supported single-arm row (p. 119) | 8-10 reps each side | 1, 1, 5 | 5 | | |
| Single-arm reverse fly (p. 121) | 10-12 reps each side | No eccentric or isometric hold | 4 (perform as a circuit with the next 2 exercises) | | Perform with single arm. |
| Half-kneeling single-arm pull-down (p. 130) | 10-12 reps each side | 1, 1, 3 | 4 | | Perform as half-kneeling. |
| Dumbbell biceps curl (p. 124) | 10-12 reps | 1, 1, 3 | 4 | | |
| **Weeks 5-8** | | | | | |
| **Warm-up/activation** | | | | | |
| Deadbug (p. 54) | 10 reps each side | No eccentric or isometric hold | 2 (perform as a circuit with the next 3 exercises) | | |
| High goblet carry (p. 46) | About 40 steps | No eccentric or isometric hold | 2 | | |

| Exercise | Reps/time | Tempo | Sets | Exercise photo | Notes |
|---|---|---|---|---|---|
| Active hang (p. 49) | 15-30 sec | No eccentric or isometric hold | 2 | | |
| Prone back extension (p. 148) | 15 reps | No eccentric or isometric hold | 2 | | |
| **Upper-body pull** | | | | | |
| Assisted neutral or supinated grip pull-up or chin-up (p. 128) | 5-8 reps (or max reps) | 1, 1, 5 | 5 (perform as a superset with the next exercise, resting 2 min between rounds) | | |
| Supported single-arm row (p. 119) | 8-10 reps each side | 1, 5, 5 | 5 | | |
| Half-kneeling single-arm cable row (p. 120) | 10-12 reps each side | 1, 3, 5 | 4 (perform as a circuit with the next 2 exercises) | | Perform as half-kneeling with single arm. |
| Seated pull-down (p. 129) | 10-12 reps | 1, 3, 3 | 4 | | |
| Alternating dumbbell hammer curl (p. 125) | 10-12 reps each side | 1, 1, 5 | 4 | | Perform as alternating. |

(continued)

## Build Sculpted Muscle Program: Workout 4 *(continued)*

| Exercise | Reps/time | Tempo | Sets | Exercise photo | Notes |
|---|---|---|---|---|---|
| **Weeks 9-12** | | | | | |
| **Warm-up/activation** | | | | | |
| Deadbug (p. 54) | 10 reps each side | No eccentric or isometric hold | 2 (perform as a circuit with the next 3 exercises) | | |
| High goblet carry (p. 46) | About 40 steps | No eccentric or isometric hold | 2 | | |
| Active hang (p. 49) | 15-30 sec | No eccentric or isometric hold | 2 | | |
| Prone back extension (p. 148) | 15 reps | No eccentric or isometric hold | 2 | | |
| **Upper-body pull** | | | | | |
| Assisted neutral or pronated pull-up (p. 126) | Max reps (up to 10) | No eccentric or isometric hold | 5 (perform as a superset with the next exercise, resting 2 min between rounds) | | Add superband to assist. |
| Supported single-arm row (p. 119) | 8-10 reps each side | No eccentric or isometric hold | 5 | | |
| Reverse fly (p. 121) | 10-12 reps | No eccentric or isometric hold | 4 (perform as a circuit with the next 3 exercises) | | |

| Exercise | Reps/time | Tempo | Sets | Exercise photo | Notes |
|---|---|---|---|---|---|
| Dumbbell biceps curl (p. 124) | 10-12 reps | No eccentric or isometric hold | 4 | 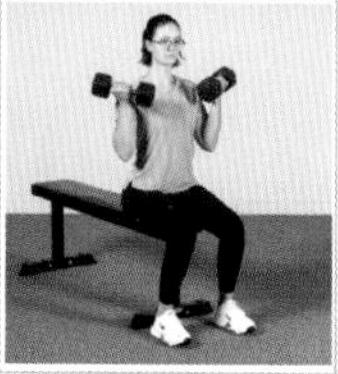 | |
| Dumbbell dynamic high pull (p. 122) | 10-12 reps | No eccentric or isometric hold | 4 | 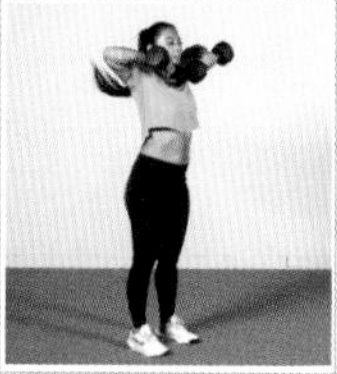 | |
| Inverted row (p. 117) | 10-12 reps | No eccentric or isometric hold | 4 | 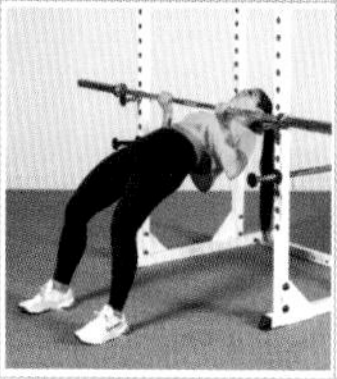 | |

## Build Sculpted Muscle Program: Workout 5

Start adding a fifth workout in week 5 of the program.

| Exercise | Reps/time | Tempo | Sets | Exercise photo | Notes |
|---|---|---|---|---|---|
| **Weeks 5-8** | | | | | |
| **Warm-up/activation** | | | | | |
| Dead hang (p. 48) | 20-30 sec | No eccentric or isometric hold | 2 (perform as a circuit with the next 4 exercises) | 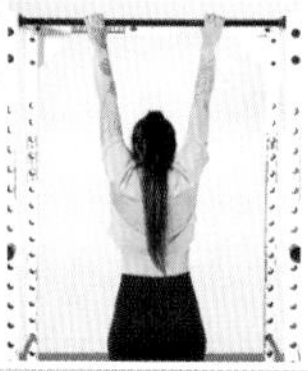 | |
| Rack carry (p. 45) | About 40 steps | No eccentric or isometric hold | 2 | 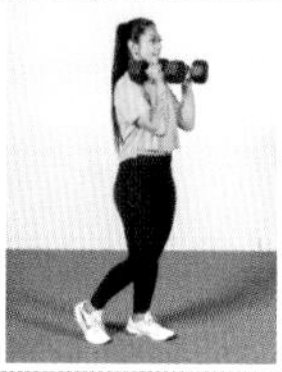 | |
| Plate pinch hold (p. 47) | 15-30 sec | No eccentric or isometric hold | 2 | 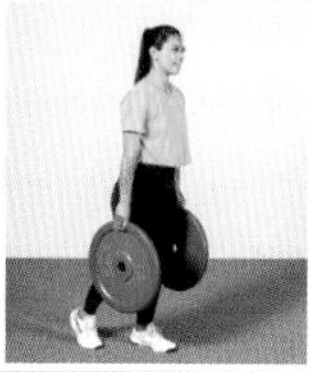 | |

*(continued)*

## Build Sculpted Muscle Program: Workout 5 *(continued)*

| Exercise | Reps/time | Tempo | Sets | Exercise photo | Notes |
|---|---|---|---|---|---|
| Standing Paloff press (p. 50) | 15 reps each side | No eccentric or isometric hold | 2 | | |
| Hollow hold (p. 60) | 15-20 sec | No eccentric or isometric hold | 2 | | |
| **Metabolic conditioning** | | | | | |
| Squat to overhead press (p. 143) | 10-12 reps | No eccentric or isometric hold | 4 (perform as a circuit with the next 4 exercises) | | |
| Cable high to low chop (p. 145) | 10-12 reps each side | X, X, 3 | 4 | | |
| Alternating plank row (p. 142) | 10-12 reps each side | No eccentric or isometric hold | 4 | | |
| Reverse lunge to dynamic lift (p. 139) | 10-12 reps each side | No eccentric or isometric hold | 4 | | |
| Copenhagen 90/90 (p. 61) | 15-30 sec each side | No eccentric or isometric hold | 4 | | |

| Exercise | Reps/time | Tempo | Sets | Exercise photo | Notes |
|---|---|---|---|---|---|
| **Weeks 9-12** | | | | | |
| **Warm-up/activation** | | | | | |
| Dead hang (p. 48) | 20-30 sec | No eccentric or isometric hold | 2 (perform as a circuit with the next 4 exercises) | | |
| Rack carry (p. 45) | About 40 steps | No eccentric or isometric hold | 2 | | |
| Plate pinch hold (p. 47) | 15-30 sec | No eccentric or isometric hold | 2 | | |
| Standing Paloff press (p. 50) | 15 reps each side | No eccentric or isometric hold | 2 | | |
| Hollow hold (p. 60) | 15-20 sec | No eccentric or isometric hold | 2 | | |
| **Metabolic conditioning** | | | | | |
| Squat to overhead press (p. 143) | 10-12 reps | No eccentric or isometric hold | 4 (perform as a circuit with the next 4 exercises) | | |
| Cable high to low chop (p. 145) | 10-12 reps each side | X, X, 3 | 4 | | |

*(continued)*

## Build Sculpted Muscle Program: Workout 5 *(continued)*

| Exercise | Reps/time | Tempo | Sets | Exercise photo | Notes |
|---|---|---|---|---|---|
| Alternating plank row (p. 142) | 10-12 reps each side | No eccentric or isometric hold | 4 | | |
| Reverse lunge to dynamic lift (p. 139) | 10-12 reps each side | No eccentric or isometric hold | 4 | | |
| Copenhagen 90/90 (p. 61) | 15-30 sec each side | No eccentric or isometric hold | 4 | | |

# 13

# GET LEAN

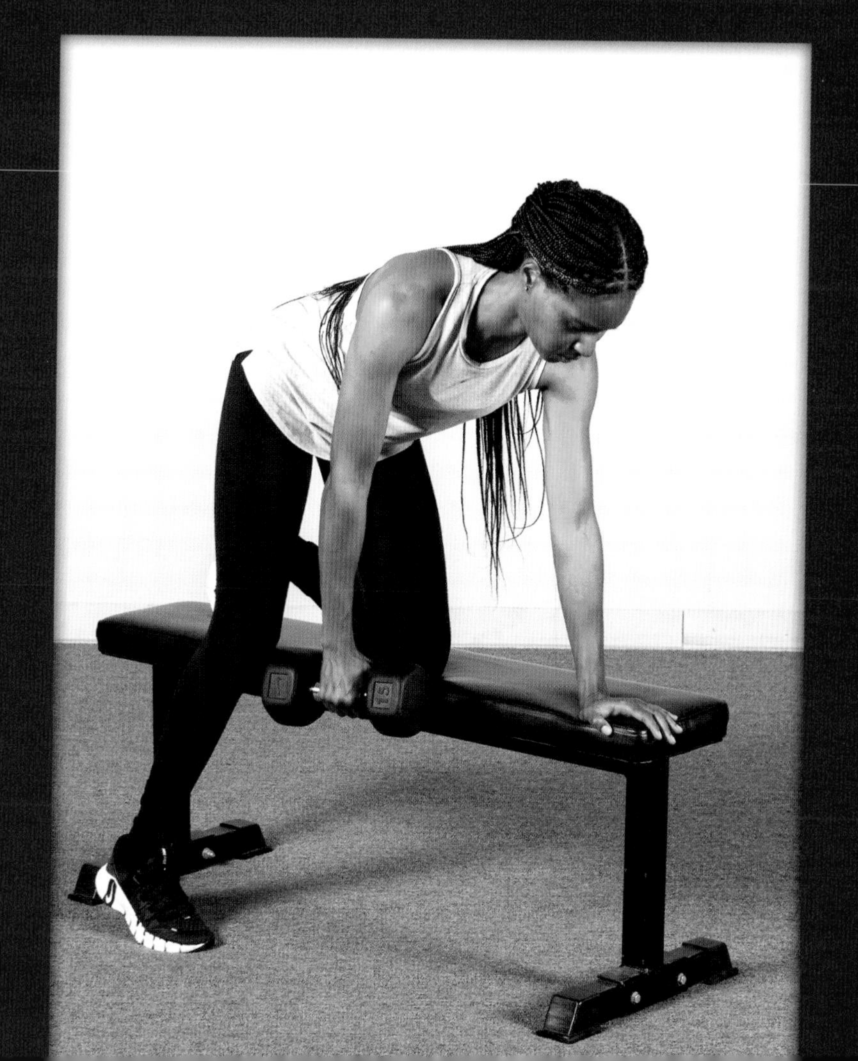

This program keeps in mind the person who loves to take classes regularly, such as dance, spin, or Pilates! It's the ideal program for someone who wants to take these classes but also do more strength training. I designed it knowing that these classes tax your body differently than a strength-training session. All three phases of this program (weeks 1-4, 5-8, and 9-12) have two workouts focused on lifting heavier weight, while the other two workouts are designed for total strength with some metabolic conditioning. This allows you to incorporate your favorite classes into your overall fitness routine. Throughout the program, you'll want to perform the exercises within each workout as a circuit (i.e., back-to-back).

*Equipment note:* The workouts in this program require a fully equipped gym, including a pull-up bar, barbell, squat rack, bench, and a variety of dumbbells.

## Get Lean Program: Workout 1

| Exercise | Reps/time | Tempo | Sets | Exercise photo | Notes |
|---|---|---|---|---|---|
| **Weeks 1-4** | | | | | |
| **Warm-up/activation** | | | | | |
| Deadbug (p. 54) | 10 reps each side | No eccentric or isometric hold | 2 (perform as a circuit with the next 3 exercises) | | |
| Body-weight squat (p. 66) | 15 reps | No eccentric or isometric hold | 2 | | Perform with body weight only. |
| Body-weight hip thrust (hold) (p. 83) | 30 sec | N/A | 2 | | Perform with body weight only. |
| Body-weight reverse lunge (p. 73) | 10 reps each side | No eccentric or isometric hold | 2 | | Perform with body weight only. |

| Exercise | Reps/time | Tempo | Sets | Exercise photo | Notes |
|---|---|---|---|---|---|
| **Heavy lower body** | | | | | |
| Goblet squat (p. 66) | 10-12 reps | 5, 1, 1 | 4 (perform as a superset with the next exercise, resting 2 min between rounds) | | |
| Barbell hip thrust (p. 83) | 10-12 reps | 1, 1, 5 | 4 | | |
| Romanian deadlift (p. 85) | 10-12 reps | 5, 1, 1 | 3 (perform as a circuit with the next 3 exercises) | | |
| Goblet stationary lunge or split squat (p. 75) | 10-12 reps each side | 5, 1, 1 | 3 | | Use goblet grip. |
| Cable abduction (p. 95) | 10-12 reps each side | No eccentric or isometric hold | 3 | | |
| Cable adduction (p. 96) | 10-12 reps each side | No eccentric or isometric hold | 3 | | |

(continued)

## Get Lean Program: Workout 1 *(continued)*

| Exercise | Reps/time | Tempo | Sets | Exercise photo | Notes |
|---|---|---|---|---|---|
| **Weeks 5-8** | | | | | |
| **Warm-up/activation** | | | | | |
| Deadbug (p. 54) | 10 reps each side | No eccentric or isometric hold | 2 (perform as a circuit with the next 3 exercises) | | |
| Body-weight squat (p. 66) | 15 reps | No eccentric or isometric hold | 2 | | Perform with body weight only. |
| Body-weight hip thrust (hold) (p. 83) | 30 sec | N/A | 2 | | Perform with body weight only. |
| Body-weight reverse lunge (p. 73) | 10 reps each side | No eccentric or isometric hold | 2 | | Perform with body weight only. |
| **Heavy lower body** | | | | | |
| Goblet squat (p. 66) | 8-10 reps each side | 5, 5, 1 | 4 (perform as a superset with the next exercise, resting 2 min between rounds) | | |
| Barbell hip thrust (p. 83) | 8-10 reps | 1, 5, 5 | 4 | | |
| Romanian deadlift (p. 85) | 10-12 reps | 5, 1, 1 | 3 (perform as a circuit with the next 3 exercises) | | |

| Exercise | Reps/time | Tempo | Sets | Exercise photo | Notes |
|---|---|---|---|---|---|
| Goblet stationary lunge or split squat (p. 75) | 10-12 reps each side | 5, 5, 1 | 3 | 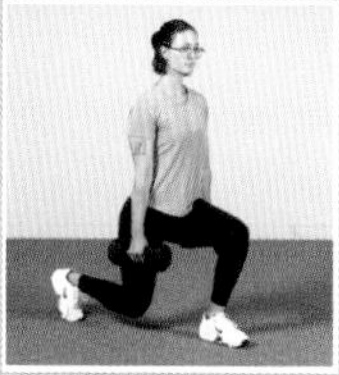 | Use goblet grip. |
| Cable abduction (p. 95) | 10-12 reps each side | No eccentric or isometric hold | 3 | 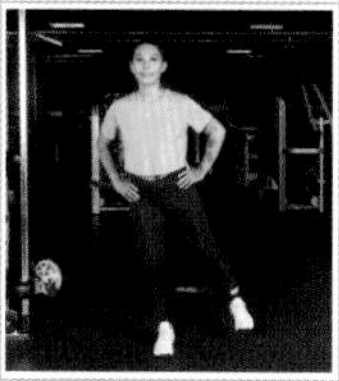 | |
| Cable adduction (p. 96) | 10-12 reps each side | No eccentric or isometric hold | 3 | 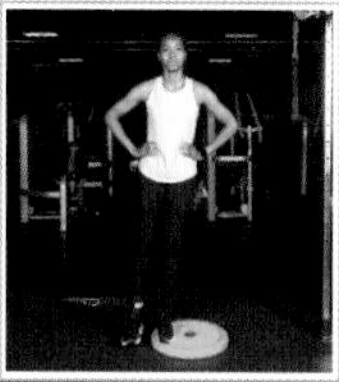 | |
| **Weeks 9-12** | | | | | |
| **Warm-up/activation** | | | | | |
| Deadbug (p. 54) | 10 reps each side | No eccentric or isometric hold | 2 (perform as a circuit with the next 3 exercises) | 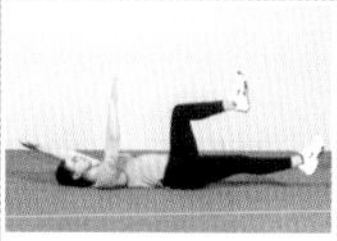 | |
| Body-weight squat (p. 66) | 15 reps | No eccentric or isometric hold | 2 | 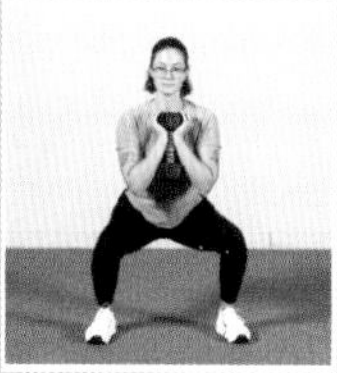 | Perform with body weight only. |
| Body-weight hip thrust (hold) (p. 83) | 30 sec | N/A | 2 | 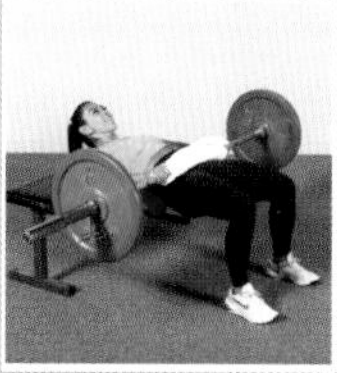 | Perform with body weight only. |
| Body-weight reverse lunge (p. 73) | 10 reps each side | No eccentric or isometric hold | 2 | 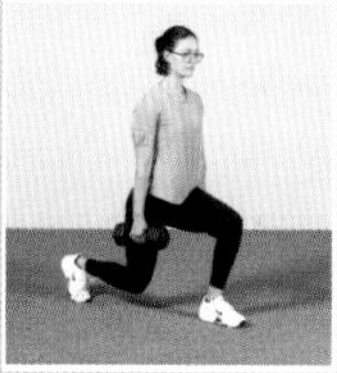 | Perform with body weight only. |

*(continued)*

## Get Lean Program: Workout 1 *(continued)*

| Exercise | Reps/time | Tempo | Sets | Exercise photo | Notes |
|---|---|---|---|---|---|
| **Heavy lower body** | | | | | |
| Front rack squat with dumbbells or barbell (p. 68) | 8-10 reps | No eccentric or isometric hold | 4 (perform as a superset with the next exercise, resting 2 min between rounds) | | |
| Barbell hip thrust (p. 83) | 8-10 reps | No eccentric or isometric hold | 4 | | |
| Romanian deadlift (p. 85) | 10-12 reps | 5, 1, 1 | 3 (perform as a circuit with the next 3 exercises) | | |
| Goblet Bulgarian split squat (p. 76) | 8-10 reps each side | No eccentric or isometric hold | 3 | | Use goblet grip. |
| Cable abduction (p. 95) | 10-12 reps each side | No eccentric or isometric hold | 3 | | |
| Cable adduction (p. 96) | 10-12 reps each side | No eccentric or isometric hold | 3 | | |

## Get Lean Program: Workout 2

| Exercise | Reps/time | Tempo | Sets | Exercise photo | Notes |
|---|---|---|---|---|---|
| Weeks 1-4 | | | | | |
| Warm-up/activation | | | | | |
| Rack carry (p. 45) | About 40 steps | No eccentric or isometric hold | 2 (perform as a circuit with the next 4 exercises) | | |
| Bird dog (p. 52) | 10 reps each side | No eccentric or isometric hold | 2 | | |
| Scapular pull-up (p. 131) | 10 reps | No eccentric or isometric hold | 2 | | |
| Prone W back extension (p. 149) | 15 reps | No eccentric or isometric hold | 2 | | |
| Forearm side plank (p. 56) | 20-30 sec each side | No eccentric or isometric hold | 2 | | |
| Heavy upper body | | | | | |
| Alternating dumbbell chest press (p. 100) | 10-12 reps each side | 1, 1, 5 | 4 (perform as a superset with the next exercise, resting 2 min between rounds) | | Perform as alternating. |

*(continued)*

## Get Lean Program: Workout 2 *(continued)*

| Exercise | Reps/time | Tempo | Sets | Exercise photo | Notes |
|---|---|---|---|---|---|
| Neutral or supinated grip pull-up/chin-up (assisted or unassisted) *or* seated pull-down with neutral or supinated grip (p. 127) | 8-10 reps (or max amount) | 1, 1, 5 | 4 | | |
| Half-kneeling overhead press (p. 106) | 10-12 reps each side | 1, 1, 5 | 3 (perform as a circuit with the next 2 exercises) | | |
| Supported single-arm row (p. 119) | 10-12 reps each side | 1, 1, 5 | 3 | | |
| Dumbbell lateral raise (p. 112) | 10-12 reps | No eccentric or isometric hold | 3 | | |
| **Weeks 5-8** | | | | | |
| **Warm-up/activation** | | | | | |
| Rack carry (p. 45) | About 40 steps | No eccentric or isometric hold | 2 (perform as a circuit with the next 4 exercises) | | |
| Deadbug (p. 54) | 10 reps each side | No eccentric or isometric hold | 2 | | |
| Scapular pull-up (p. 131) | 10 reps | No eccentric or isometric hold | 2 | | |

| Exercise | Reps/time | Tempo | Sets | Exercise photo | Notes |
|---|---|---|---|---|---|
| Prone W back extension (p. 149) | 15 reps | No eccentric or isometric hold | 2 | | |
| Forearm side plank (p. 56) | 20-30 sec each side | No eccentric or isometric hold | 2 | | |
| **Heavy upper body** | | | | | |
| Alternating dumbbell chest press (p. 100) | 10-12 reps each side | 1, 5, 5 | 4 (perform as a superset with the next exercise, resting 2 min between rounds) | | Perform as alternating. |
| Neutral or supinated grip pull-up/chin-up (assisted or unassisted) *or* seated pull-down with neutral or supinated grip (p. 127) | 8-10 reps (or max amount) | 1, 5, 5 | 4 | | |
| Alternating tall kneeling overhead press (p. 107) | 10-12 reps each side | 1, 1, 5 | 3 (perform as a circuit with the next 2 exercises) | | Perform as alternating. |
| Alternating dumbbell bent-over row (p. 118) | 10-12 reps each side | 1, 1, 5; reset after each rep if necessary | 3 | | Perform as alternating. |
| Dumbbell lateral raise (p. 112) | 10-12 reps | No eccentric or isometric hold | 3 | | |

(continued)

## Get Lean Program: Workout 2 *(continued)*

| Exercise | Reps/time | Tempo | Sets | Exercise photo | Notes |
|---|---|---|---|---|---|
| **Weeks 9-12** | | | | | |
| **Warm-up/activation** | | | | | |
| Rack carry (p. 45) | About 40 steps | No eccentric or isometric hold | 2 (perform as a circuit with the next 4 exercises) | | |
| Deadbug (p. 54) | 10 reps each side | No eccentric or isometric hold | 2 | | |
| Scapular pull-up (p. 131) | 10 reps | No eccentric or isometric hold | 2 | | |
| Prone W back extension (p. 149) | 15 reps | No eccentric or isometric hold | 2 | | |
| Forearm side plank (p. 56) | 20-30 sec each side | No eccentric or isometric hold | 2 | | |
| **Heavy upper body** | | | | | |
| Dumbbell chest press (p. 100) | 8-10 reps | No eccentric or isometric hold | 4 (perform as a superset with the next exercise, resting 2 min between rounds) | | |

| Exercise | Reps/time | Tempo | Sets | Exercise photo | Notes |
|---|---|---|---|---|---|
| Neutral or supinated grip pull-up/chin-up (assisted or unassisted) *or* seated pull-down with neutral or supinated grip (p. 127) | 8-10 reps (or max amount) | No eccentric or isometric hold | 4 | 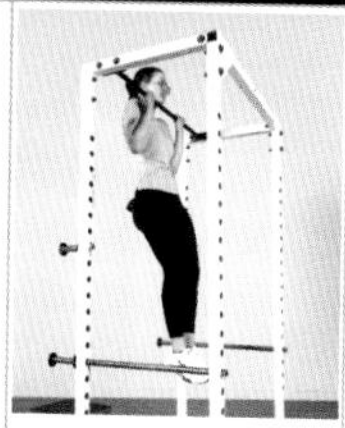 | |
| Tall kneeling overhead press (p. 107) | 8-10 reps | No eccentric or isometric hold | 3 (perform as a circuit with the next 2 exercises) | 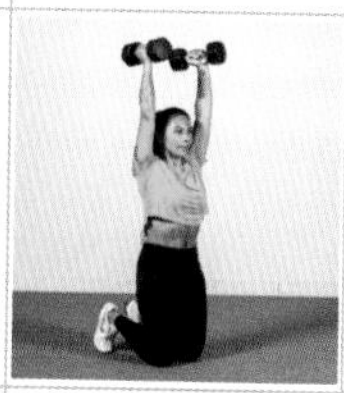 | |
| Inverted row (p. 117) | 8-10 reps | No eccentric or isometric hold | 3 | 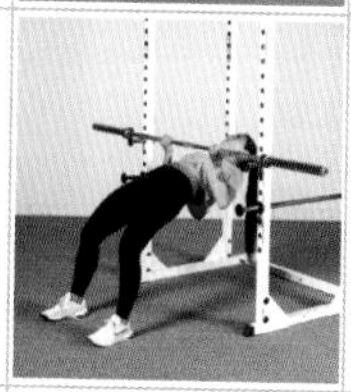 | |
| Dumbbell lateral raise + dumbbell front raise alternating combo (p. 112, 111) | 8-10 reps each | No eccentric or isometric hold | 3 | 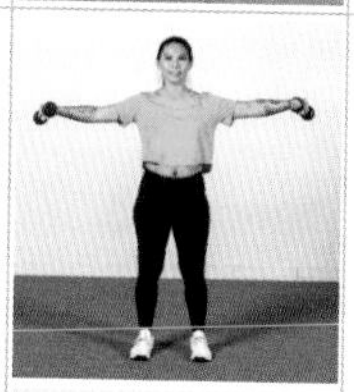 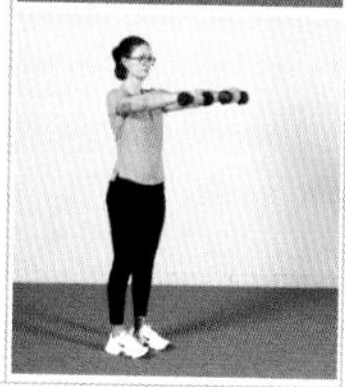 | |

## Get Lean Program: Workout 3

| Exercise | Reps/time | Tempo | Sets | Exercise photo | Notes |
|---|---|---|---|---|---|
| Weeks 1-4 | | | | | |
| **Warm-up/activation** | | | | | |
| Deadbug (p. 54) | 10 reps each side | No eccentric or isometric hold | 2 (perform as a circuit with the next 3 exercises) | | |
| Shoulder tap (p. 59) | 10 reps each side | No eccentric or isometric hold | 2 | | |
| Staggered Paloff press (p. 51) | 10 reps each side | No eccentric or isometric hold | 2 | | |
| Suitcase carry (p. 44) | About 20 steps each side | No eccentric or isometric hold | 2 | | |
| **Total body conditioning** | | | | | |
| Alternating plank row (p. 142) | 12-15 reps each side | No eccentric or isometric hold | 4 (perform as a circuit with the next 3 exercises, resting 2 min between rounds) | | |
| Squat to overhead press (p. 143) | 12-15 reps | No eccentric or isometric hold | 4 | | |

| Exercise | Reps/time | Tempo | Sets | Exercise photo | Notes |
|---|---|---|---|---|---|
| Dumbbell dynamic high pull (p. 122) | 12-15 reps | No eccentric or isometric hold | 4 | | |
| Run or incline walk on treadmill or cycling intervals (p. 156) | 3 rounds of 30 sec with 30 sec rest in between | N/A | 4 | | |
| **Weeks 5-8** | | | | | |
| **Warm-up/activation** | | | | | |
| Deadbug (p. 54) | 10 reps each side | No eccentric or isometric hold | 2 (perform as a circuit with the next 3 exercises) | | |
| Shoulder tap (p. 59) | 10 reps each side | No eccentric or isometric hold | 2 | | |
| Staggered Paloff press (p. 51) | 10 reps each side | No eccentric or isometric hold | 2 | | |
| Suitcase carry (p. 44) | About 20 steps each side | No eccentric or isometric hold | 2 | | |

*(continued)*

## Get Lean Program: Workout 3 *(continued)*

| Exercise | Reps/time | Tempo | Sets | Exercise photo | Notes |
|---|---|---|---|---|---|
| **Total body conditioning** | | | | | |
| Squat to row (p. 147) | 12-15 reps | No eccentric or isometric hold | 4 (perform as a circuit with the next 3 exercises, resting 2 min between rounds) | | |
| Dumbbell push press (p. 109) | 12-15 reps | No eccentric or isometric hold | 4 | | |
| Cable high to low chop (p. 145) | 12-15 reps each side | No eccentric or isometric hold | 4 | | |
| Run or incline walk on treadmill or cycling intervals (p. 156) | 3 rounds of 30 sec with 30 sec rest in between | N/A | 4 | | |
| **Weeks 9-12** | | | | | |
| **Warm-up/activation** | | | | | |
| Deadbug (p. 54) | 10 reps each side | No eccentric or isometric hold | 2 (perform as a circuit with the next 3 exercises) | | |
| Shoulder tap (p. 59) | 10 reps each side | No eccentric or isometric hold | 2 | | |

| Exercise | Reps/time | Tempo | Sets | Exercise photo | Notes |
|---|---|---|---|---|---|
| Staggered Paloff press (p. 51) | 10 reps each side | No eccentric or isometric hold | 2 | | |
| Suitcase carry (p. 44) | About 20 steps each side | No eccentric or isometric hold | 2 | | |
| **Total body conditioning** | | | | | |
| Squat to overhead press (p. 143) | 12-15 reps | No eccentric or isometric hold | 4 (perform as a circuit with the next 3 exercises, resting 2 min between rounds) | | |
| Dumbbell clean (p. 123) | 12-15 reps | No eccentric or isometric hold | 4 | | |
| Reverse lunge to dynamic lift (p. 139) | 12-15 reps each side | No eccentric or isometric hold | 4 | | |
| Run or incline walk on treadmill or cycling intervals (p. 156) | 3 rounds of 30 sec with 30 sec rest in between | N/A | 4 | | |

## Get Lean Program: Workout 4

| Exercise | Reps/time | Tempo | Sets | Exercise photo | Notes |
|---|---|---|---|---|---|
| Weeks 1-4 | | | | | |
| **Warm-up/activation** | | | | | |
| Rack carry (p. 45) | About 40 steps | No eccentric or isometric hold | 2 (perform as a circuit with the next 3 exercises) | | |
| Prone back extension (p. 148) | 15 reps | No eccentric or isometric hold | 2 | | |
| Body-weight hip thrust (p. 83) | 15 reps | No eccentric or isometric hold | 2 | | Perform with body weight only. |
| Hollow hold (p. 60) | 15-20 sec | No eccentric or isometric hold | 2 | | |
| **Total body conditioning** | | | | | |
| Dumbbell bent-over row (p. 118) | 12-15 reps | No eccentric or isometric hold | 4 (perform as a circuit with the next 4 exercises, resting 2 min between rounds) | | |
| Single-leg bridge (p. 82) | 12-15 reps each side | No eccentric or isometric hold | 4 | | |
| Staggered cable twist (p. 146) | 12-15 reps each side | No eccentric or isometric hold | 4 | | |

| Exercise | Reps/time | Tempo | Sets | Exercise photo | Notes |
|---|---|---|---|---|---|
| Dumbbell or body-weight step-up (p. 77) | 12-15 reps each side | No eccentric or isometric hold | 4 | | Start with body weight; stay on same side. |
| Run or incline walk on treadmill or cycling intervals (p. 156) | 3 rounds of 30 sec with 30 sec rest in between | N/A | 4 | | |
| **Weeks 5-8** | | | | | |
| **Warm-up/activation** | | | | | |
| Rack carry (p. 45) | About 40 steps | No eccentric or isometric hold | 2 (perform as a circuit with the next 3 exercises) | | |
| Prone back extension (p. 148) | 15 reps | No eccentric or isometric hold | 2 | | |
| Body-weight hip thrust (p. 83) | 15 reps | No eccentric or isometric hold | 2 | | Perform with body weight only. |
| Hollow hold (p. 60) | 15-20 sec | No eccentric or isometric hold | 2 | | |

(continued)

## Get Lean Program: Workout 4 *(continued)*

| Exercise | Reps/time | Tempo | Sets | Exercise photo | Notes |
|---|---|---|---|---|---|
| **Total body conditioning** | | | | | |
| Cable plank pull (p. 150) | 12-15 reps each side | No eccentric or isometric hold | 4 (perform as a circuit with the next 4 exercises, resting 2 min between rounds) | | |
| Long bridge (p. 82) | 12-15 reps | No eccentric or isometric hold | 4 | | |
| Standing low to high lift (p. 135) | 12-15 reps each side | No eccentric or isometric hold | 4 | | |
| Alternating dumbbell or body-weight step-up (p. 77) | 12-15 reps each side | No eccentric or isometric hold | 4 | | Start with body weight. |
| Run or incline walk on treadmill or cycling intervals (p. 156) | 3 rounds of 30 sec with 30 sec rest in between | N/A | 4 | | |
| **Weeks 9-12** | | | | | |
| **Warm-up/activation** | | | | | |
| Rack carry (p. 45) | About 40 steps | No eccentric or isometric hold | 2 (perform as a circuit with the next 3 exercises) | | |
| Prone back extension (p. 148) | 15 reps | No eccentric or isometric hold | 2 | | |

| Exercise | Reps/time | Tempo | Sets | Exercise photo | Notes |
|---|---|---|---|---|---|
| Body-weight hip thrust (p. 83) | 15 reps | No eccentric or isometric hold | 2 | | Perform with body weight only. |
| Hollow hold (p. 60) | 15-20 sec | No eccentric or isometric hold | 2 | | |
| **Total body conditioning** | | | | | |
| Squat to row (p. 147) | 12-15 reps | No eccentric or isometric hold | 4 (perform as a circuit with the next 4 exercises, resting 2 min between rounds) | | |
| Dumbbell bridge (p. 81) | 12-15 reps | No eccentric or isometric hold | 4 | | |
| Cable high to low chop (p. 145) | 12-15 reps each side | No eccentric or isometric hold | 4 | | |
| Alternating dumbbell or body-weight step-up (p. 77) | 12-15 reps each side | No eccentric or isometric hold | 4 | | Start with body weight. |
| Run or incline walk on treadmill *or* cycling intervals (p. 156) | 3 rounds of 30 sec with 30 sec rest in between | N/A | 4 | | |

# 14

# IMPROVE MUSCLE ENDURANCE

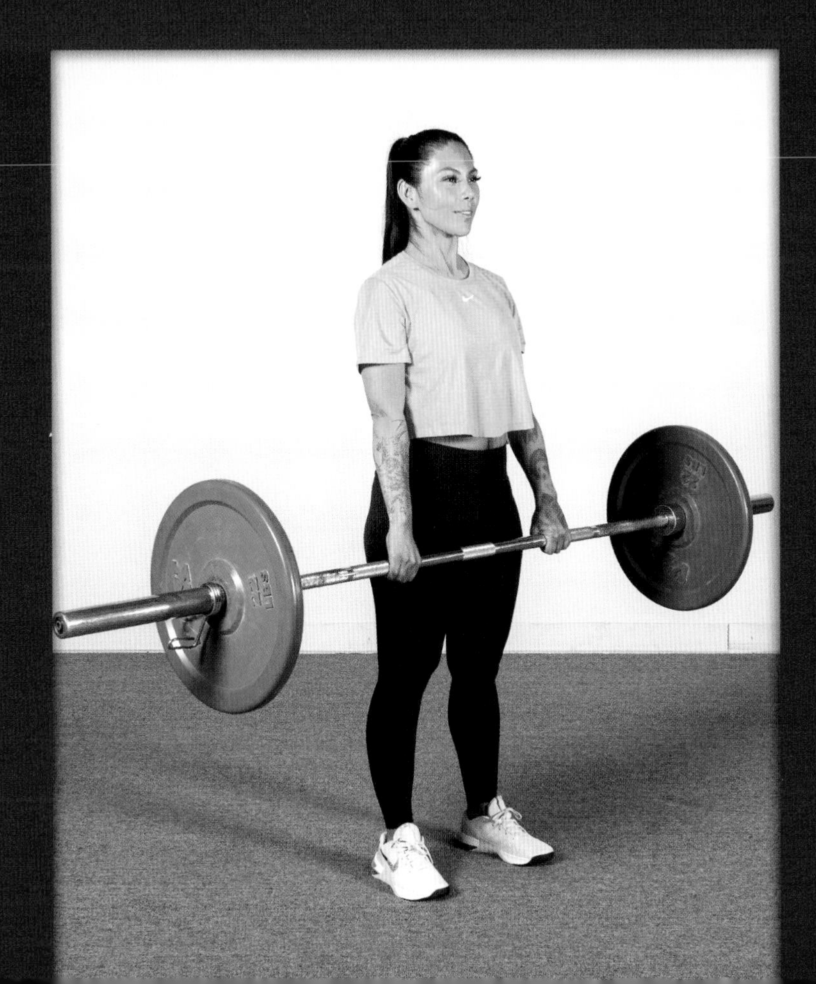

This strength program is created for someone who wants to move better, longer, and stronger. I designed the workouts to move in multiple planes, knowing this would be ideal for someone who plays sports regularly. There are 4 workouts for each of the three phases (weeks 1-4, 5-8, and 9-12), with two focused on heavier lifting. The other two are a combination of total body strength and conditioning. Of course, recreational sports can be tough on your body, so feel free to let a match or game stand in for one or both of the total body workouts. Throughout the program, you'll want to perform the exercises within each workout as a circuit (i.e., back-to-back). You can do this program at home or in a small gym, as long as you have the right equipment (see the following note).

*Equipment note:* The workouts in this program require a range of dumbbells (5-45 pounds), a cable machine or superband, a treadmill or stationary bike, and a bench. A barbell and weight plates are optional.

## Improve Muscle Endurance Program: Workout 1

| Exercise | Reps/time | Tempo | Sets | Exercise photo | Notes |
|---|---|---|---|---|---|
| **Weeks 1-4** | | | | | |
| **Warm-up/activation** | | | | | |
| Deadbug (p. 54) | 10 reps each side | No eccentric or isometric hold | 2 (perform as a circuit with the next 3 exercises) | | |
| Body-weight squat (p. 66) | 15 reps | No eccentric or isometric hold | 2 | | Perform with body weight only. |
| Body-weight hip thrust (hold) (p. 83) | 30 sec | No eccentric or isometric hold | 2 | | Perform with body weight only. |
| Body-weight reverse lunge (p. 73) | 10 reps each side | No eccentric or isometric hold | 2 | | Perform with body weight only. |

| Exercise | Reps/time | Tempo | Sets | Exercise photo | Notes |
|---|---|---|---|---|---|
| | | **Heavy lower body** | | | |
| Goblet squat (p. 66) | 10-12 reps | 5, 1, 1 | 4 (perform as a superset with the next exercise, resting 2 min between rounds) | | |
| Barbell or dumbbell hip thrust (p. 83) | 10-12 reps | 1, 1, 5 | 4 | | Start with dumbbells. |
| Romanian deadlift (p. 85) | 10-12 reps | 5, 1, 1 | 3 (perform as a circuit with the next 3 exercises) | | |
| Goblet stationary lunge or split squat (p. 75) | 10-12 reps each side | 5, 1, 1 | 3 | | Use goblet grip. |
| Side-lying abduction (p. 93) | 10-12 reps each side | No eccentric or isometric hold | 3 | | |
| Side-lying hip circles (p. 92) | 10-12 reps each direction and side | No eccentric or isometric hold | 3 | | |

*(continued)*

## Improve Muscle Endurance Program: Workout 1 *(continued)*

| Exercise | Reps/time | Tempo | Sets | Exercise photo | Notes |
|---|---|---|---|---|---|
| **Weeks 5-8** | | | | | |
| **Warm-up/activation** | | | | | |
| Deadbug (p. 54) | 10 reps each side | No eccentric or isometric hold | 2 (perform as a circuit with the next 3 exercises) | | |
| Body-weight squat (p. 66) | 15 reps | No eccentric or isometric hold | 2 | | Perform with body weight only. |
| Body-weight hip thrust (hold) (p. 83) | 30 sec | N/A | 2 | | Perform with body weight only. |
| Body-weight reverse lunge (p. 73) | 10 reps each side | No eccentric or isometric hold | 2 | | Perform with body weight only. |
| **Heavy lower body** | | | | | |
| Goblet squat (p. 66) | 8-10 reps each side | 5, 5, 1 | 4 (perform as a superset with the next exercise, resting 2 min between rounds) | | |
| Barbell or dumbbell hip thrust (p. 83) | 8-10 reps | 5, 5, 1 | 4 | | Start with dumbbells. |
| Romanian deadlift (p. 85) | 10-12 reps | 5, 1, 1 | 3 (perform as a circuit with the next 3 exercises) | | |
| Goblet stationary lunge or split squat (p. 75) | 10-12 reps each side | 5, 5, 1 | 3 | | Use goblet grip. |

| Exercise | Reps/time | Tempo | Sets | Exercise photo | Notes |
|---|---|---|---|---|---|
| Side-lying abduction (p. 93) | 10-12 reps each side | No eccentric or isometric hold | 3 | | |
| Side-lying hip circles (p. 92) | 10-12 reps each direction and side | No eccentric or isometric hold | 3 | | |
| **Weeks 9-12** | | | | | |
| **Warm-up/activation** | | | | | |
| Deadbug (p. 54) | 10 reps each side | No eccentric or isometric hold | 2 (perform as a circuit with the next 3 exercises) | | |
| Body-weight squat (p. 66) | 15 reps | No eccentric or isometric hold | 2 | | Perform with body weight only. |
| Body-weight hip thrust (hold) (p. 83) | 30 sec | No eccentric or isometric hold | 2 | | Perform with body weight only. |
| Body-weight reverse lunge (p. 73) | 10 reps each side | No eccentric or isometric hold | 2 | | Perform with body weight only. |

*(continued)*

## Improve Muscle Endurance Program: Workout 1 *(continued)*

| Exercise | Reps/time | Tempo | Sets | Exercise photo | Notes |
|---|---|---|---|---|---|
| | | **Heavy lower body** | | | |
| Front squat with dumbbells (p. 69) | 8-10 reps | No eccentric or isometric hold | 4 (perform as a superset with the next exercise, resting 2 min between rounds) | 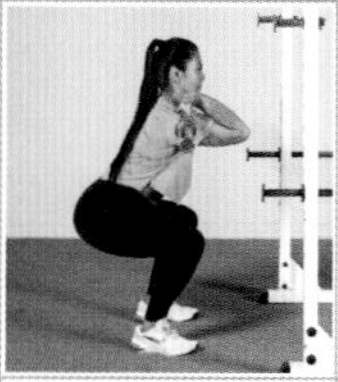 | Use dumbbells. |
| Single-leg bridge (p. 82) | 8-10 reps each side | No eccentric or isometric hold | 4 | 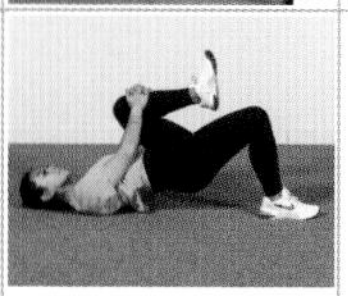 | |
| Romanian deadlift (p. 85) | 10-12 reps | No eccentric or isometric hold | 3 (perform as a circuit with the next 3 exercises) | 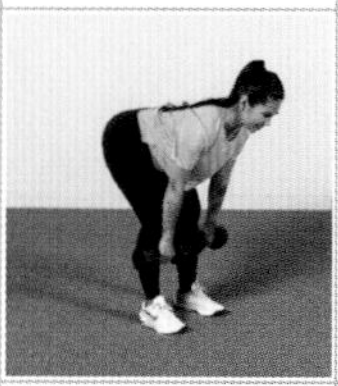 | |
| Goblet Bulgarian split squat (p. 76) | 8-10 reps each side | No eccentric or isometric hold | 3 | 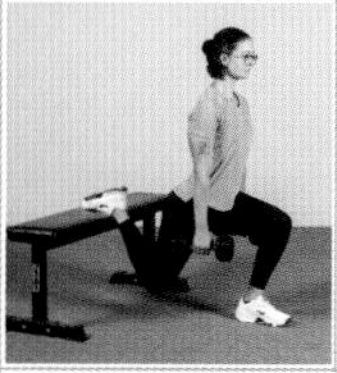 | Use goblet grip. |
| Side-lying abduction (p. 93) | 10-12 reps each side | No eccentric or isometric hold | 3 | 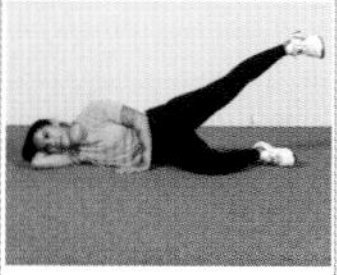 | |
| Side-lying hip circles (p. 92) | 10-12 reps each direction and side | No eccentric or isometric hold | 3 | 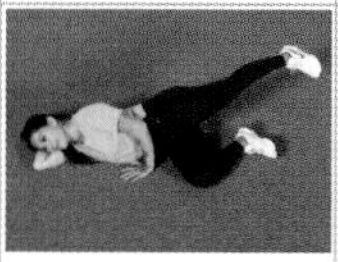 | |

## Improve Muscle Endurance Program: Workout 2

| Exercise | Reps/time | Tempo | Sets | Exercise photo | Notes |
|---|---|---|---|---|---|
| **Weeks 1-4** | | | | | |
| **Warm-up/activation** | | | | | |
| Rack carry (p. 45) | About 40 steps | No eccentric or isometric hold | 2 (perform as a circuit with the next 3 exercises) | | |
| Bird dog (p. 52) | 10 reps each side | No eccentric or isometric hold | 2 | | |
| Prone W back extension (p. 149) | 15 reps | No eccentric or isometric hold | 2 | | |
| Forearm side plank (p. 56) | 20-30 sec each side | No eccentric or isometric hold | 2 | | |
| **Heavy upper body** | | | | | |
| Alternating dumbbell chest press (p. 100) | 10-12 reps each side | 1, 1, 5 | 4 (perform as a superset with the next exercise, resting 2 min between rounds) | | Perform as alternating. |
| Supported single-arm row (p. 119) | 10-12 reps each side | 1, 1, 5 | 4 | | |
| Half-kneeling overhead press (p. 106) | 10-12 reps each side | 1, 1, 5 | 3 (perform as a circuit with the next 3 exercises) | | |

(continued)

## Improve Muscle Endurance Program: Workout 2 *(continued)*

| Exercise | Reps/time | Tempo | Sets | Exercise photo | Notes |
|---|---|---|---|---|---|
| Dumbbell biceps curl (p. 124) | 10-12 reps | 1, 1, 5 | 3 | | |
| Single-arm reverse fly (p. 121) | 10-12 reps each side | 1, 1, 5 | 3 | | Perform with single arm. |
| Dumbbell lateral raise (p. 112) | 10-12 reps | No eccentric or isometric hold | 3 | | |
| **Weeks 5-8** | | | | | |
| **Warm-up/activation** | | | | | |
| Rack carry (p. 45) | About 40 steps | No eccentric or isometric hold | 2 (perform as a circuit with the next 3 exercises) | | |
| Deadbug (p. 54) | 10 reps each side | No eccentric or isometric hold | 2 | | |
| Prone W back extension (p. 149) | 15 reps | No eccentric or isometric hold | 2 | | |
| Forearm side plank (p. 56) | 20-30 sec each side | No eccentric or isometric hold | 2 | | |

| Exercise | Reps/time | Tempo | Sets | Exercise photo | Notes |
|---|---|---|---|---|---|
| **Heavy upper body** | | | | | |
| Alternating dumbbell chest press (p. 100) | 10-12 reps each side | 1, 5, 5 | 4 (perform as a superset with the next exercise, resting 2 min between rounds) | 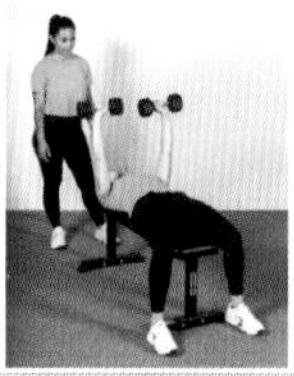 | Perform as alternating. |
| Supported single-arm row (p. 119) | 10-12 reps each side | 1, 5, 5 | 4 | 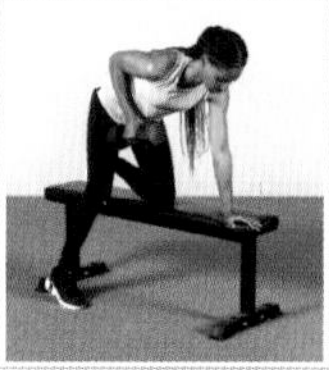 | |
| Alternating tall kneeling overhead press (p. 107) | 10-12 reps each side | 1, 1, 5 | 3 (perform as a circuit with the next 3 exercises) | 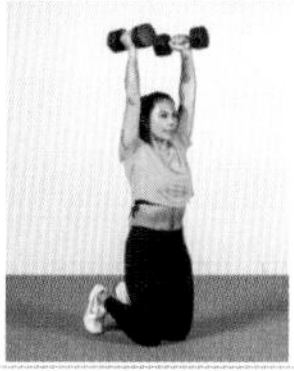 | Perform as alternating. |
| Dumbbell hammer curl (p. 125) | 10-12 reps each side | 1, 1, 5 | 3 | 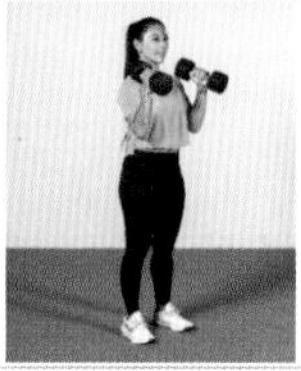 | |
| Single-arm reverse fly (p. 121) | 10-12 reps each side | No eccentric or isometric hold | 3 | 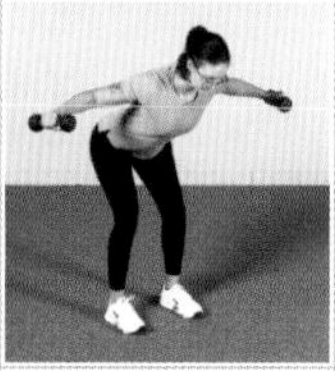 | Perform with single arm. |
| Dumbbell lateral raise (p. 112) | 10-12 reps | No eccentric or isometric hold | 3 | 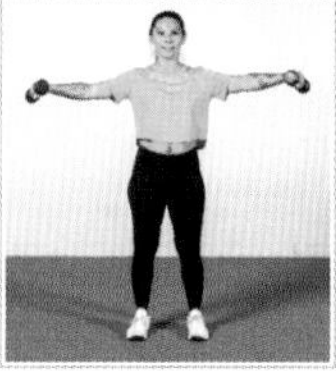 | |

(continued)

## Improve Muscle Endurance Program: Workout 2 *(continued)*

| Exercise | Reps/time | Tempo | Sets | Exercise photo | Notes |
|---|---|---|---|---|---|
| **Weeks 9-12** | | | | | |
| **Warm-up/activation** | | | | | |
| Rack carry (p. 45) | About 40 steps | No eccentric or isometric hold | 2 (perform as a circuit with the next 3 exercises) | 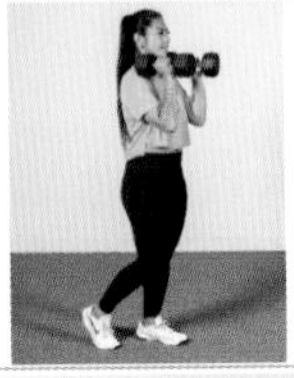 | |
| Deadbug (p. 54) | 10 reps each side | No eccentric or isometric hold | 2 | 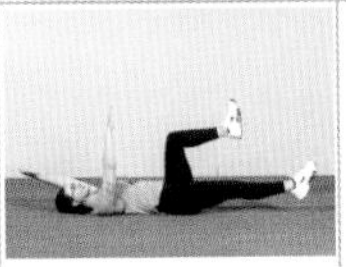 | |
| Prone W back extension (p. 149) | 15 reps | No eccentric or isometric hold | 2 | 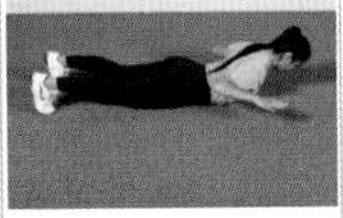 | |
| Forearm side plank (p. 56) | 20-30 sec each side | No eccentric or isometric hold | 2 | 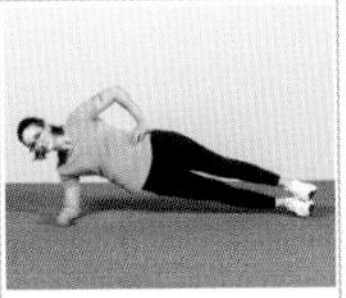 | |
| **Heavy upper body** | | | | | |
| Dumbbell chest press (p. 100) | 8-10 reps | No eccentric or isometric hold | 4 (perform as a superset with the next exercise, resting 2 min between rounds) | 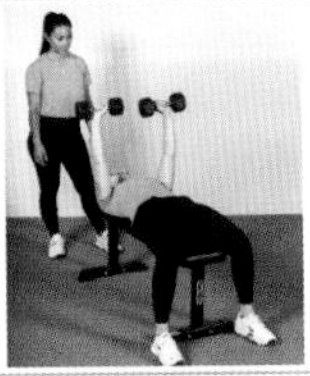 | |
| Dumbbell bent-over row (p. 118) | 8-10 reps | No eccentric or isometric hold | 4 | 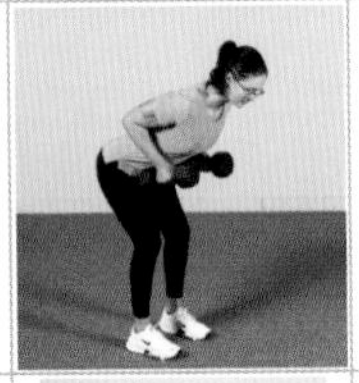 | |
| Tall kneeling overhead press (p. 107) | 8-10 reps | No eccentric or isometric hold | 3 (perform as a circuit with the next 3 exercises) | 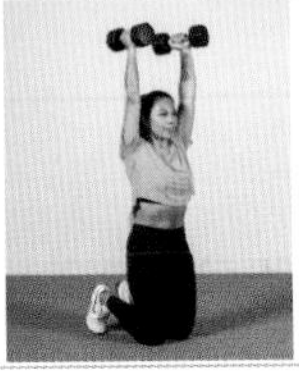 | |

| Exercise | Reps/time | Tempo | Sets | Exercise photo | Notes |
|---|---|---|---|---|---|
| Biceps curl and hammer curl alternating combo (p. 124-125) | 8-10 reps each | No eccentric or isometric hold | 3 | 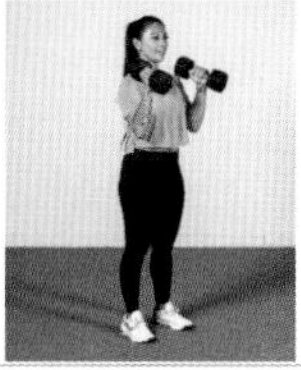 | |
| Reverse fly (p. 121) | 8-10 reps | No eccentric or isometric hold | 3 | 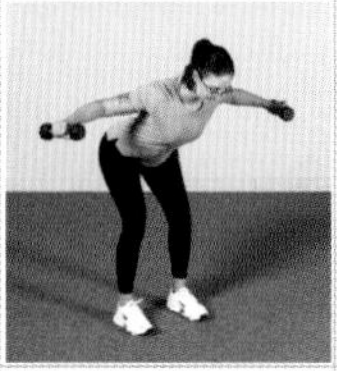 | |
| Dumbbell lateral raise + dumbbell front raise alternating combo (p. 112, 111) | 8-10 reps each | No eccentric or isometric hold | 3 | 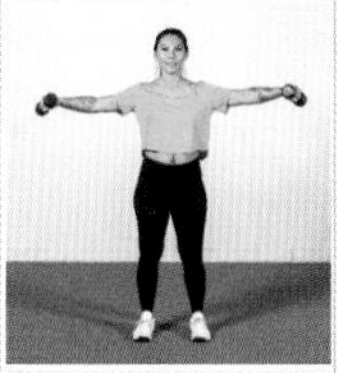 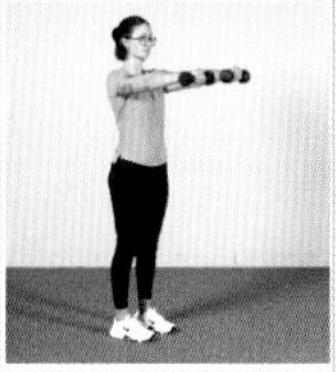 | |

## Improve Muscle Endurance Program: Workout 3

| Exercise | Reps/time | Tempo | Sets | Exercise photo | Notes |
|---|---|---|---|---|---|
| **Weeks 1-4** | | | | | |
| **Warm-up/activation** | | | | | |
| Deadbug (p. 54) | 10 reps each side | No eccentric or isometric hold | 2 (perform as a circuit with the next 3 exercises) | | |
| Shoulder tap (p. 59) | 10 reps each side | No eccentric or isometric hold | 2 | | |
| Staggered Paloff press (p. 51) | 10 reps each side | No eccentric or isometric hold | 2 | | |
| Suitcase carry (p. 44) | About 20 steps each side | No eccentric or isometric hold | 2 | | |
| **Total body conditioning** | | | | | |
| Rotational overhead press (p. 140) | 12-15 reps each side | No eccentric or isometric hold | 4 (perform as a circuit with the next 4 exercises, resting 2 min between rounds) | | |
| Goblet stationary lateral lunge (p. 78) | 12-15 reps each side | No eccentric or isometric hold | 4 | | Use goblet grip. |
| Alternating plank row (p. 142) | 12-15 reps each side | No eccentric or isometric hold | 4 | | |

| Exercise | Reps/time | Tempo | Sets | Exercise photo | Notes |
|---|---|---|---|---|---|
| Copenhagen 90/90 (p. 61) | 15-30 sec | No eccentric or isometric hold | 4 | | |
| Run or incline walk on treadmill or cycling intervals (p. 156) | 3 rounds of 30 sec with 30 sec rest in between | N/A | 4 | | |
| **Weeks 5-8** | | | | | |
| **Warm-up/activation** | | | | | |
| Deadbug (p. 54) | 10 reps each side | No eccentric or isometric hold | 2 (perform as a circuit with the next 3 exercises) | | |
| Shoulder tap (p. 59) | 10 reps each side | No eccentric or isometric hold | 2 | | |
| Staggered Paloff press (p. 51) | 10 reps each side | No eccentric or isometric hold | 2 | | |
| Suitcase carry (p. 44) | About 20 steps each side | No eccentric or isometric hold | 2 | | |
| **Total body conditioning** | | | | | |
| Alternating step back to curl and press (p. 141) | 10-12 reps each side | No eccentric or isometric hold | 4 (perform as a circuit with the next 4 exercises, resting 2 min between rounds) | | |

*(continued)*

## Improve Muscle Endurance Program: Workout 3 *(continued)*

| Exercise | Reps/time | Tempo | Sets | Exercise photo | Notes |
|---|---|---|---|---|---|
| Alternating goblet lateral lunge (p. 78) | 12-15 reps each side | No eccentric or isometric hold | 4 | | Use goblet grip. |
| Alternating plank row (p. 142) | 10-12 reps each side | No eccentric or isometric hold | 4 | | |
| Copenhagen 90/90 (p. 61) | 15-30 sec | No eccentric or isometric hold | 4 | | |
| Run or incline walk on treadmill *or* cycling intervals (p. 156) | 3 rounds of 30 sec with 30 sec rest in between | N/A | 4 | | |
| **Weeks 9-12** | | | | | |
| **Warm-up/activation** | | | | | |
| Deadbug (p. 54) | 10 reps each side | No eccentric or isometric hold | 2 (perform as a circuit with the next 3 exercises) | | |
| Shoulder tap (p. 59) | 10 reps each side | No eccentric or isometric hold | 2 | | |
| Staggered Paloff press (p. 51) | 10 reps each side | No eccentric or isometric hold | 2 | | |
| Suitcase carry (p. 44) | About 20 steps each side | No eccentric or isometric hold | 2 | | |

| Exercise | Reps/time | Tempo | Sets | Exercise photo | Notes |
|---|---|---|---|---|---|
| **Total body conditioning** | | | | | |
| Rotational overhead press (p. 140) | 10-12 reps each side | No eccentric or isometric hold | 4 (perform as a circuit with the next 4 exercises, resting 2 min between rounds) | | |
| Alternating goblet back diagonal lunge (p. 80) | 10-12 reps each side | No eccentric or isometric hold | 4 | | Use goblet grip. |
| Alternating plank row (p. 142) | 10-12 reps each side | No eccentric or isometric hold | 4 | | |
| Copenhagen 90/90 (p. 61) | 15-30 sec | No eccentric or isometric hold | 4 | | |
| Run or incline walk on treadmill or cycling intervals (p. 156) | 3 rounds of 30 sec with 30 sec rest in between | N/A | 4 | | |

## Improve Muscle Endurance Program: Workout 4

| Exercise | Reps/time | Tempo | Sets | Exercise photo | Notes |
|---|---|---|---|---|---|
| **Weeks 1-4** | | | | | |
| **Warm-up/activation** | | | | | |
| High rack carry (p. 45) | About 40 steps | No eccentric or isometric hold | 2 (perform as a circuit with the next 3 exercises) | 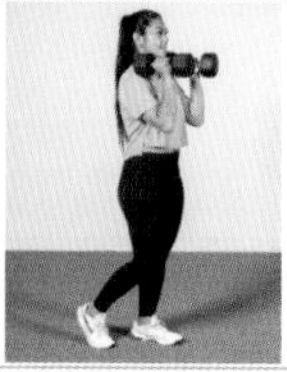 | Use high rack position: even with the ears. |
| Prone back extension (p. 148) | 15 reps | No eccentric or isometric hold | 2 | 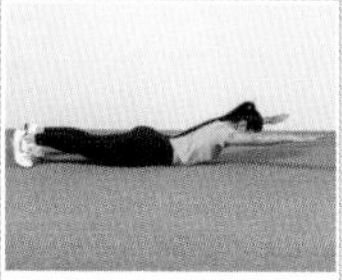 | |
| Body-weight hip thrust (p. 83) | 15 reps | No eccentric or isometric hold | 2 | 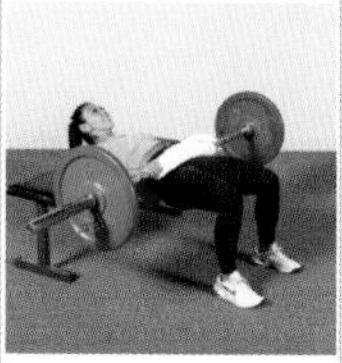 | Perform with body weight only. |
| Hollow hold (p. 60) | 15-20 sec | No eccentric or isometric hold | 2 | 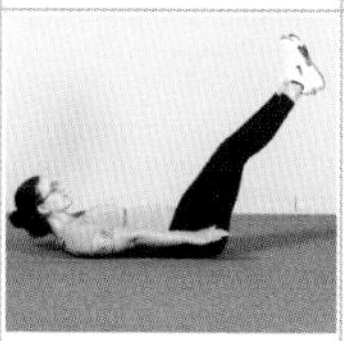 | |
| **Total body conditioning** | | | | | |
| Squat to row (p. 147) | 12-15 reps | No eccentric or isometric hold | 4 (perform as a circuit with the next 4 exercises, resting 2 min between rounds) | 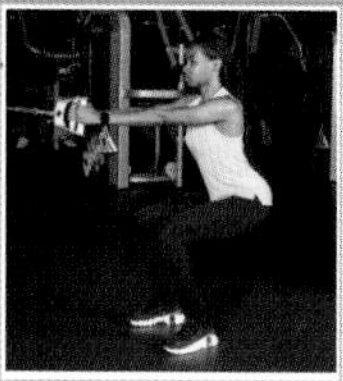 | |
| Staggered barbell or body-weight hip thrust (p. 84) | 12-15 reps each side | 5, 5, 1 | 4 | 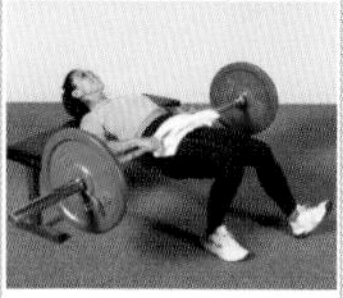 | Start with body weight. |
| Goblet staggered squat (p. 70) | 12-15 reps each side | No eccentric or isometric hold | 4 | 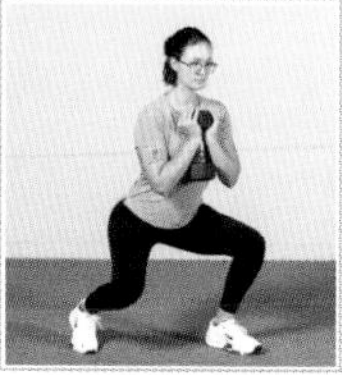 | |

| Exercise | Reps/time | Tempo | Sets | Exercise photo | Notes |
|---|---|---|---|---|---|
| Hinge to row rotation (p. 144) | 12-15 reps each side | No eccentric or isometric hold | 4 | | |
| Run or incline walk on treadmill or cycling intervals (p. 156) | 3 rounds of 30 sec with 30 sec rest in between | N/A | 4 | | |
| **Weeks 5-8** | | | | | |
| **Warm-up/activation** | | | | | |
| High rack carry (p. 45) | About 40 steps | No eccentric or isometric hold | 2 (perform as a circuit with the next 3 exercises) | | Use high rack position: even with the ears. |
| Prone back extension (p. 148) | 15 reps | No eccentric or isometric hold | 2 | | |
| Body-weight hip thrust (p. 83) | 15 reps | No eccentric or isometric hold | 2 | | Perform with body weight only. |
| Hollow hold (p. 60) | 15-20 sec | No eccentric or isometric hold | 2 | | |

*(continued)*

## Improve Muscle Endurance Program: Workout 4 *(continued)*

| Exercise | Reps/time | Tempo | Sets | Exercise photo | Notes |
|---|---|---|---|---|---|
| | | **Total body conditioning** | | | |
| Cable plank pull (p. 150) | 12-15 reps each side | No eccentric or isometric hold | 4 (perform as a circuit with the next 4 exercises, resting 2 min between rounds) | 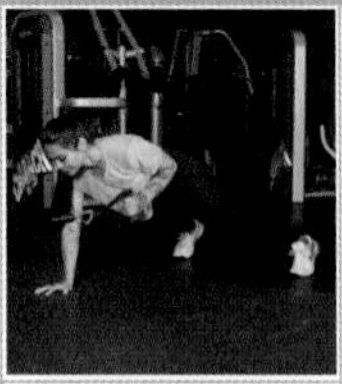 | |
| Single-leg bridge (p. 82) | 12-15 reps | 5, 5, 1 | 4 | 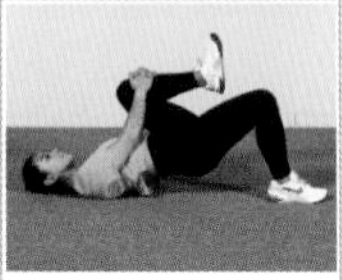 | |
| Dumbbell curtsy lunge (p. 79) | 12-15 reps each side | No eccentric or isometric hold | 4 | 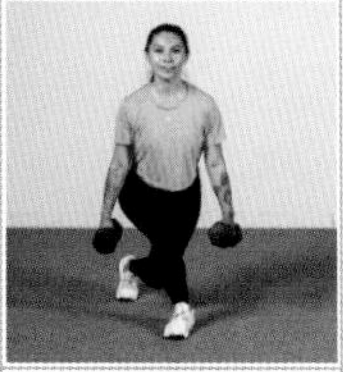 | Stay on same side. |
| Dumbbell dynamic high pull (p. 122) | 12-15 reps | No eccentric or isometric hold | 4 | 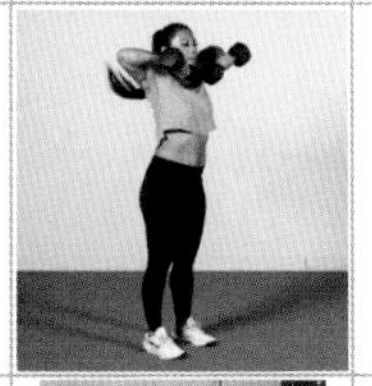 | |
| Run or incline walk on treadmill or cycling intervals (p. 156) | 3 rounds of 30 sec with 30 sec rest in between | N/A | 4 | 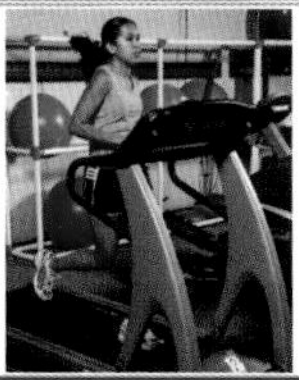 | |
| | | **Weeks 9-12** | | | |
| | | **Warm-up/activation** | | | |
| High rack carry (p. 45) | About 40 steps | No eccentric or isometric hold | 2 (perform as a circuit with the next 3 exercises) | 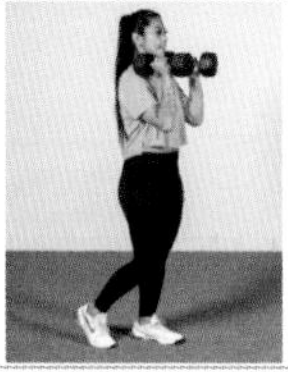 | Use high rack position: even with the ears. |
| Prone back extension (p. 148) | 15 reps | No eccentric or isometric hold | 2 | 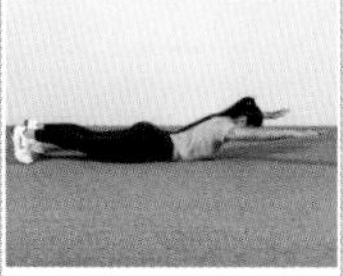 | |

| Exercise | Reps/time | Tempo | Sets | Exercise photo | Notes |
|---|---|---|---|---|---|
| Body-weight hip thrust (p. 83) | 15 reps | No eccentric or isometric hold | 2 | | Perform with body weight only. |
| Hollow hold (p. 60) | 15-20 sec | No eccentric or isometric hold | 2 | | |
| **Total body conditioning** | | | | | |
| Cable plank pull (p. 150) | 12-15 reps each side | No eccentric or isometric hold | 4 (perform as a circuit with the next 4 exercises, resting 2 min between rounds) | | |
| Dumbbell long bridge (p. 82) | 12-15 reps | No eccentric or isometric hold | 4 | | Perform with dumbbells. |
| Alternating dumbbell curtsy lunge (p. 79) | 12-15 reps each side | No eccentric or isometric hold | 4 | | |
| Dumbbell clean (p. 123) | 12-15 reps | No eccentric or isometric hold | 4 | | |
| Run or incline walk on treadmill *or* cycling intervals (p. 156) | 3 rounds of 30 sec with 30 sec rest in between | N/A | 4 | | |

# ABOUT THE AUTHOR

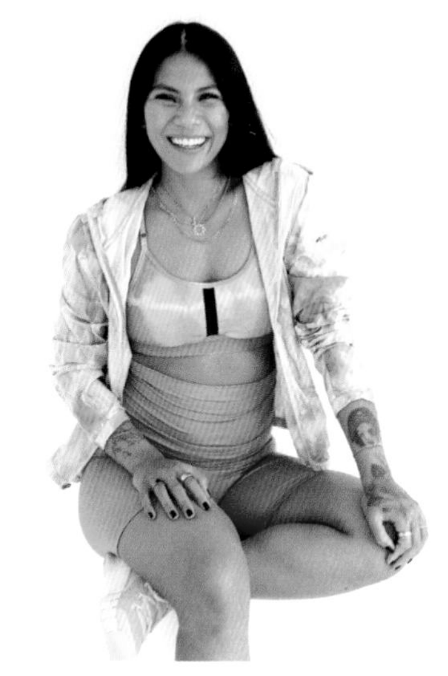
Amber Tice Photography

**Betina Gozo Shimonek** has over a decade of experience as a certified trainer. She has worked for over 10 years as a Nike Global Trainer, programming and consulting for the brand, and she was featured in the Nike Training Club app leading a popular Strength for Beginners program. In 2016, she won the *Women's Health* Next Fitness Star contest. She published *The Woman's Guide to Strength Training* in 2017. She also partnered with *Prevention* magazine in 2019 to create *Get Strong With Betina Gozo*, a four-week workout DVD for beginners and aging people who want to stay active.

Gozo Shimonek cohosts the lifestyle podcast *Beyond the Routine* alongside her husband, Nic. They also created an accessible performance training platform, LiNE UP With Us. She was one of the original 21 trainers featured on the Apple Fitness+ team, teaching weekly strength and core workouts and leading the service's Workouts for Beginners program. She is also a contributor to the Nike Well Collective, which focuses on five pillars of holistic fitness: movement, mindfulness, nutrition, rest, and connection.

Gozo Shimonek is passionate about empowering women to work out in any stage of their lives. From killer workouts to tips on how to navigate the weight room, she shares her expertise to help women get the most out of their resistance workouts. She also travels the world, empowering and connecting women through her women's-only strength training workshops and women's strength training camps.

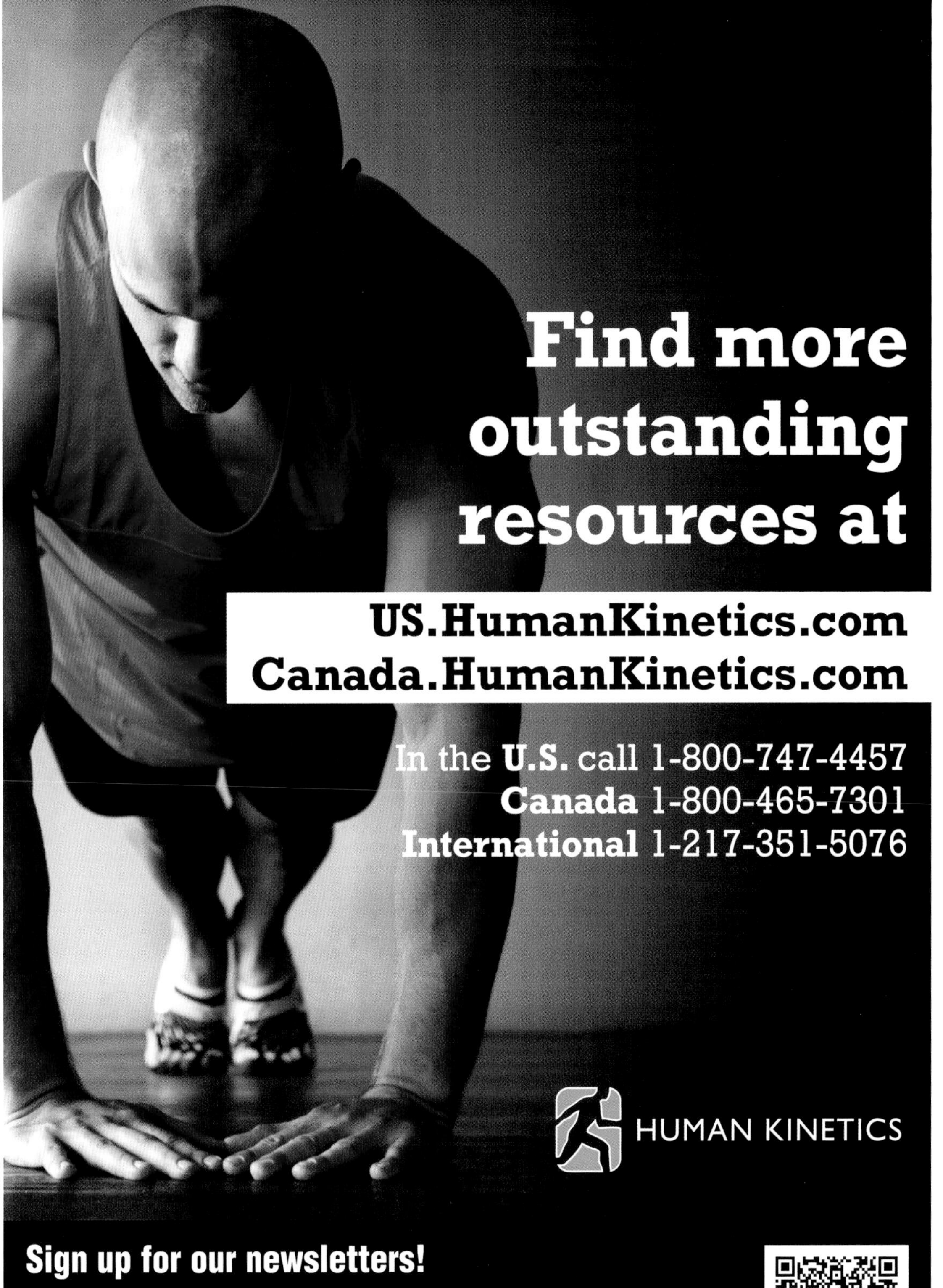


**Sign up for our newsletters!**

Get the latest insights with regular newsletters, plus periodic product information and special insider offers from Human Kinetics.